MCQs
for the
MRCP Part 1

The MRCP (Part 2) Postgraduate Training Series has been compiled by the University of Wales College of Medicine. The 38 video tapes concentrate on the short-cases examination and will help candidates avoid the common pitfalls.

Astra Pharmaceuticals Ltd recognize the importance of continuing medical education and are the sponsors of this video training series.

If you are preparing for the MRCP (Part 2) exam, and would like to view the tapes, please contact:
    The Continuing Medical Education Dept.
    Astra Pharmaceuticals Limited
    Home Park
    Kings Langley
    Herts
    WD4 8DH

MCQs for the MRCP Part 1

by

Mark Sanderson MRCP(UK) **(Editor)**
Registrar in Public Health Medicine, Fulbourn Hospital,
Cambridge;
formerly Registrar in General and Respiratory Medicine,
Guy's Hospital, London

Dennis Barnes MRCP(UK)
Research Registrar in Metabolic Medicine, United Medical
and Dental Schools of Guy's and St Thomas',
Guy's Hospital, London

Michael Polkey MRCP(UK)
Registrar in General and Respiratory Medicine,
Guy's Hospital, London

Andrew Winrow MRCP(UK)
Senior Registrar in Paediatrics,
St Mary's Hospital, London

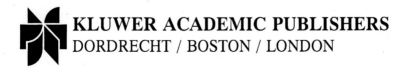
KLUWER ACADEMIC PUBLISHERS
DORDRECHT / BOSTON / LONDON

Distributors

---

for the United States and Canada: Kluwer Academic Publishers, PO Box 358,
Accord Station, Hingham, MA 02018-0358, USA
for all other countries: Kluwer Academic Publishers Group, Distribution Center,
PO Box 322, 3300 AH Dordrecht, The Netherlands

ISBN 0-7923-8834-8

A catalogue record for this book is available from the British Library.

Copyright

Published in the United Kingdom by Kluwer Academic Publishers, PO Box 55,
Lancaster, UK.

Kluwer Academic Publishers BV incorporates the publishing programmes of D. Reidel,
Martinus Nijhoff, Dr W. Junk and MTP Press.

Printed and bound in Great Britain by Cromwell Press, Melksham, Wilts.

Contents

Introduction

The MRCP(UK) examination is now sat by many candidates at several sites throughout the world; the diploma is eagerly sought by those who wish to undertake a variety of careers as well as those who aspire to become physicians or paediatricians. As a result this examination has attracted a large volume of books and other teaching aids to assist the candidate in his or her preparation. We would like to add our contribution to this area.

From October 1993, the Colleges will be offering Part 1 papers in General Medicine and Paediatrics. Both papers will have a common 30 questions, the remainder covering the particular specialty. We therefore felt it would be appropriate to cover both areas in this book. However, we have not tried to reproduce the exact structure of the examinations, but offer two papers on General Medicine and one on Paediatrics.

An important part of revision based around self-testing with MCQs is the explanation of some of the answers and the follow-up of those areas where an individual's knowledge is a bit vague! We therefore provide short summaries with each set of answers followed by up-to-date references. We hope that you find this helpful in your revision programme.

I would like to thank my co-authors for all their hard work, Ben Green for checking through the questions and Jackie Bradley for typing some of the initial draft.

Mark Sanderson
May 1993

Section 1 – General Medicine

1. The following statements regarding the complications of strokes are correct:

A. cerebral haemorrhage may be complicated by the syndrome of inappropriate ADH secretion
B. cerebral oedema associated with cerebral haemorrhage should be treated with corticosteroids
C. secondary haemorrhagic transformation is a common complication of cardioembolic stroke
D. aspiration pneumonia more commonly complicates brainstem strokes as opposed to unilateral hemispheric strokes
E. in the management of acute stroke, attempts should be made to keep blood pressure below 180/100 by using short-acting anti-hypertensive agents

2. Acute pancreatitis:

A. is idiopathic in more than 60% of cases
B. is a recognized side-effect of carbamazepine therapy
C. may be caused by ascariasis
D. secondary to alcohol has a higher mortality rate than for gallstone-associated pancreatitis
E. is a risk factor for the development of pancreatic carcinoma

3. The following are recognised causes of pulmonary disease:

A. nebulised pentamidine
B. amiodarone
C. sulphasalazine
D. oral contraceptives
E. aspirin

1

4. **The following are true of connective tissue disorders:**

A. both arterial and venous thromboses may occur in the antiphospholipid antibody syndrome

B. in more than 90% of patients with antiphospholipid antibodies, lupus anticoagulant will also be present

C. in severe lupus nephritis, patients with recently diagnosed systemic lupus erythematosus who present with an abrupt deterioration of renal function have a worse prognosis than those with a more chronic course

D. plasmapheresis is the treatment of choice for severe lupus nephritis

E. in patients with renal transplants for the treatment of lupus nephritis, recurrence of the condition in the allograft is extremely common

5. **The following statements are true regarding plasma lipids and diabetes mellitus:**

A. poor glycaemic control in non-insulin-dependent diabetes is associated with elevation in plasma triglycerides

B. good glycaemic control in insulin-dependent diabetes is associated with reduction in plasma HDL cholesterol

C. weight reduction in obese non-insulin-dependent diabetic subjects tends to increase plasma HDL

D. anion-exchange resins are the first line of treatment when there is elevation of both LDL cholesterol and triglycerides

E. when the nephrotic syndrome is caused by diabetes, both plasma cholesterol and triglycerides are increased

6. **Concerning iron metabolism in adults:**

A. total body stores are about 20 g

B. each pregnancy 'consumes' about 3 g

C. absorption is inhibited by coffee

D. the principal storage site is the intestinal mucosa

E. the principal method of absorption is diffusion

7. The following are true of cytokines:

A. they are a group of compounds produced exclusively by activated macrophages
B. they are exclusively polypeptides
C. they are implicated in the pathogenesis of asthma
D. they are responsible for producing a fever in infection
E. they include endotoxin as an example

8. Mitral valve prolapse:

A. is more common in younger women than older women
B. rarely causes chest pain
C. is not a factor for infective endocarditis
D. can lead to cerebral emboli
E. rarely requires mitral valve replacement

9. The following are true of testicular tumours:

A. 80% of germ cell tumours are seminomas
B. testicular maldescent is a risk factor for the development of germ cell tumours
C. most patients with teratomas have raised serum concentrations of α-fetoprotein or chorionic gonadotrophin, or both
D. back pain is a recognised presentation
E. they may metastasise to the mediastinum and occur in association with acute myeloid leukaemia

10. **The neuroleptic malignant syndrome:**

A. has been reported with the use of phenothiazines but not butyrophenones
B. typically presents with the acute development of fever, muscle rigidity, altered consciousness and autonomic dysfunction in patients on neuroleptics
C. may be complicated by seizures
D. is often associated with markedly elevated serum creatinine levels at presentation
E. may respond to bromocriptine therapy

11. **In normal ageing the following occur:**

A. there is evidence of declining T lymphocyte function
B. there are fewer taste buds
C. prolongation of the PR interval of the ECG
D. declining creatinine clearance
E. loss of voluntary muscle fibres

12. **Legionnaire's disease:**

A. is a notifiable disease in England and Wales
B. affects males more commonly than females
C. normally occurs in outbreaks
D. has a similar mortality to Pontiac fever
E. can be caught from whirlpools

13. **Raynaud's phenomenon:**

A. classically manifests with cyanosis of the digits, followed by pallor and rubor
B. may be provoked by chemicals
C. may be a feature of hypothyroidism
D. should be treated by cervical sympathectomy if medical treatment has failed
E. may be improved if the patient stops smoking

14. Hyperglycaemic hyperosmolar non-ketotic coma:

A. may be a presenting feature of diabetes mellitus
B. should be treated with a less rigorous fluid replacement regimen and with a higher dose of intravenous insulin compared with the management of ketoacidosis
C. is often fatal because of associated cerebral oedema
D. has a better prognosis than coma secondary to diabetic ketoacidosis
E. is an indication for long-term insulin therapy in the majority of patients

15. Concerning phosphorous metabolism:

A. absorption is primarily in the colon
B. reduced dietary intake causes an increase in calcitriol
C. renal excretion is not affected until the GFR is less than 30 ml/min
D. it is not important to treat hyperphosphataemia in dialysis patients
E. custard has a high phosphate content

16. Misuse of 'ecstasy' (3,4-methylenedioxymetamphetamine) is known to cause:

A. jaundice
B. disseminated intravascular coagulation (DIC)
C. rhabdomyolysis
D. trismus
E. malignant carcinoid syndrome

17. A loud first heart sound is a feature of:

A.   first-degree heart block
B.   mitral stenosis
C.   short PR interval
D.   tachycardia (in general)
E.   pericardial effusion

18. In the investigation of possible Cushing's syndrome:

A.   circadian rhythm of plasma free cortisol as measured by radioimmunoassay is a common screening test
B.   concomitant rifampicin therapy may lead to an increase in false positive dexamethasone suppression tests
C.   an insulin tolerance test may be helpful in distinguishing Cushing's syndrome from pseudo-Cushing's syndrome due to depressive illness
D.   heart failure may be associated with loss of circadian rhythm of plasma cortisol
E.   measurement of corticotrophin-releasing hormone (CRH) may be helpful in cases of Cushing's syndrome secondary to an ectopic CRH source

19. In central retinal artery occlusion:

A.   visual loss is certain after 75 minutes
B.   there is an association with migraine
C. CO_2 rebreathing is recommended
D.   mitral valve prolapse is not a recognised association
E.   the finding of an ESR of 115 mm/h would not influence management

20. The following drugs are recognised causes of constipation:

A. frusemide
B. calcium carbonate
C. vincristine
D. dipyridamole
E. cimetidine

21. Regarding *Pneumocystis carinii* pneumonia (PCP):

A. it occurs only in patients with AIDS
B. when the causative organism, may be cultured in mice
C. prophylaxis is indicated in all HIV+ patients
D. it often presents with a pleural effusion
E. prognosis may be improved with steroid therapy

22. Antineutrophil cytoplasmic antibodies (ANCA) are:

A. found in 5% of healthy people
B. exclusively IgG antibodies
C. found with increased frequency in ulcerative colitis
D. able to enter the interior of granulocytes
E. a useful diagnostic test in Wegener's granulomatosis

23. The following are true of thyroid function tests:

A. non-thyroidal illness causes a reduction in the peripheral conversion of T4 to T3
B. corticosteroids suppress TSH secretion
C. free T4 is the most reliable indicator of thyroid function during pregnancy
D. patients on combined oral contraceptive therapy have a lower free T4 concentration because of increased thyroid binding globulin levels
E. amiodarone-induced hyperthyroidism may be associated with normal total T4 concentrations

24. Sideroblastic anaemia may occur in:

A. alcohol abuse
B. mercury poisoning
C. myelodysplastic syndromes
D. patients on chloramphenicol therapy
E. infectious mononucleosis

25. The following are non-parametric statistical tests:

A. Wilcoxon's rank sum tests
B. chi-squared
C. Student's t
D. Mann–Whitney
E. Nemars

26. Intravenous magnesium:

A. causes vasodilatation of both the coronary and peripheral circulation
B. slows down conduction through the atrioventricular node
C. is absolutely contraindicated in renal failure
D. has been shown to improve morbidity but not mortality in the short term when given to patients with suspected acute myocardial infarction
E. is frequently used in the treatment of severe hypercalcaemia

27. Octreotide:

A. is a somatostatin antagonist
B. inhibits ACTH secretion
C. is more effective than pituitary surgery in the treatment of acromegaly
D. may cause gallstones
E. has been used in the treatment of variceal bleeding

28. In Parkinson's disease:

A. vertical gaze palsy suggests that there will be a good response to L-dopa therapy
B. symptoms appear when nigrostriatal dopamine falls to 50% of normal
C. Lewy bodies are pathognomonic of Parkinson's disease
D. selegiline is a useful treatment
E. the tremor frequency is usually about 25 Hz

29. The following are true of gallstones:

A. pigment stones may occur in thalassaemia
B. oestrogens may cause gallstones
C. in the over 60s, gallstones are commoner in men than women
D. the majority of patients with gallbladder cancer also have gallstones
E. calcified gallstones may be dissolved using methyl *tert*-butyl ether

30. Brucellosis:

A. is rare in Europe
B. is contracted by the bite of infected sheep
C. is a recognised cause of epididymo-orchitis
D. can be contracted from the cattle vaccine
E. has an incubation period of 1–3 weeks

31. The following statements concerning gout are correct:

A. gout is unusual in women prior to the menopause
B. gout may be associated with hereditary renal tubular disorders
C. tophi may occur in Heberden nodes
D. the dose of allopurinol needs to be reduced in renal impairment to avoid toxicity
E. allopurinol may cause a vasculitis

32. Human insulin:

A. differs from porcine insulin by one amino acid residue
B. is absorbed more quickly than porcine insulin when given subcutaneously
C. should not be given in combination with either sulphonylureas or metformin
D. has been shown to be associated with greater loss of awareness of hypoglycaemia compared with animal insulins in most double-blind randomised crossover studies
E. is more likely to cause recurrent severe hypoglycaemia in patients with tight diabetic control compared with their poorly controlled counterparts

33. Microalbuminuria:

A. is defined as the passage of small particles of albumin in urine which is not otherwise detectable by Albustix
B. is a predictor of death from cardiovascular disease only in the diabetic population
C. in an insulin-dependent diabetic patient is almost always associated with proliferative retinopathy
D. has been shown to be significantly reduced by strict glycaemic control in insulin-dependent diabetic patients
E. is present in 30% of patients with newly diagnosed insulin-dependent diabetes mellitus

34. The following skin disorders can be seen more frequently in people who abuse alcohol:

A. psoriasis
B. discoid eczema
C. pityriasis versicolor
D. rosacea
E. porphyria cutanea tarda

35. In the management of chronic heart failure:

A. secondary to severe aortic stenosis, balloon valvuloplasty often provides long-lasting symptomatic relief
B. ACE inhibitors are the only vasodilators which have been shown to improve survival
C. metolazone is useful as adjunctive therapy because it is a potent loop diuretic
D. angio-oedema may be an adverse effect of ACE inhibitors
E. long-term digoxin therapy has been shown to provide symptomatic relief only in patients with atrial fibrillation

36. Hyperprolactinaemia:

A. may be a cause of primary amenorrhoea
B. may be caused by hyperthyroidism
C. when associated with a prolactinoma, should be monitored by regular serum prolactin estimations during pregnancy to screen for tumour expansion
D. when associated with a macroprolactinoma should be treated surgically rather than medically
E. is a cause of impotence

37. Serotonin (5HT):

A. has specific receptor sites in the cerebral arteries
B. has the same effect as sumitriptan
C. release is blocked by the use of methylene dioxymethamphetamine (MDMA; 'ecstasy')
D. antagonists are antiemetics
E. levels are high in depression

38. Alcohol-induced liver cirrhosis:

A.   is a decreasing cause of death
B.   is more likely to follow regular than binge drinking (assuming consumption of an equal total)
C.   may give a similar histological appearance to that produced by amiodarone
D.   has a 60% 5-year survival if the patient abstains
E.   is associated with aminoaciduria

39. In primary pulmonary hypertension:

A.   hypertrophy of the media of small pulmonary arteries is a typical finding
B.   plexiform vascular lesions are associated with a good prognosis
C.   pulmonary artery pressure is elevated in advanced disease
D.   heart/lung transplantation is contraindicated
E.   vasodilators may be useful

40. Urticarial vasculitis:

A.   may be associated with Sjögren's syndrome
B.   may be precipitated by alcohol
C.   is often accompanied by high serum complement levels
D.   is recognised histologically by a leucocytoclastic vasculitis
E.   usually responds well to antihistamine alone

41. Phaeochromocytoma:

A.   is the second commonest cause of endocrine hypertension
B.   is a malignant condition in approximately 30% of cases
C.   may present with sudden unexplained cardiac decompensation
D.   is sometimes treated with metaiodobenzylguanidine (MIBG)
E.   may present with hypotension rather than hypertension

42. In adult idiopathic thrombocytopenic purpura:

A. men are more often affected than women
B. marrow megakaryocytes are increased
C. platelet-specific IgA can be demonstrated
D. splenectomy is the treatment of choice
E. if the patient is pregnant, the fetus can also be affected

43. When drowning:

A. salt water causes alveolar collapse whereas fresh water leads to intact (albeit fluid filled) alveoli
B. the rescued ocean swimmer is often intravascularly depleted
C. continuous positive airway pressure (CPAP) is a useful technique in resuscitation
D. corticosteroids are helpful
E. everybody aspirates water

44. In narcolepsy:

A. there is a 98% incidence of HLA-DR2 and HLA-DQwl antigens
B. acromegaly is more common
C. muscular weakness induced by laughing would be unusual
D. abnormalities of REM sleep are observed
E. dextroamphetamine is a useful treatment

45. Malaria:

A. can be acquired congenitally
B. severity is proportional to the percentage parasitaemia
C. may be treated with quinidine
D. may be complicated by Gram-negative septicaemia
E. cannot occur in individuals who have never left the UK

46. In Behçet's disease:

A.   presentation occurs most commonly in the fifth to sixth decade
B.   renal impairment is common
C.   dural sinus thrombosis may occur
D.   myocardial infarction is a recognised complication
E.   thalidomide is effective in the treatment of severe recurrent aphthous stomatitis

47. Fasting hypoglycaemia:

A.   may occur in Addison's disease
B.   with very high plasma insulin and C-peptide levels, and mildly elevated plasma proinsulin concentration are characteristic findings of an insulinoma
C.   due to sulphonylurea ingestion is confirmed by elevation of insulin, C-peptide and proinsulin of similar magnitude
D.   may be caused by antiinsulin antibodies
E.   may be due to the secretion of IGF-II by tumours

48. In renovascular hypertension:

A.   isotope renography will identify 70% of renal artery stenoses
B.   due to atherosclerosis, renal failure is an uncommon consequence in the elderly population
C.   successful treatment of the hypertension by angioplasty is more likely to occur in cases of fibromuscular dysplasia rather than atherosclerosis
D.   the ratio of peripheral to renal renin activity is a useful predictor of outcome in patients who are being considered for vascular reconstruction
E.   loop diuretics are particularly useful in the medical management

49. In status epilepticus:

A. jerking movements may cease altogether
B. cerebral blood flow is increased
C. intracranial pressure falls
D. pancreatitis is a recognised complication
E. seizures may be allowed to continue for up to 90 minutes before proceeding to general anaesthesia

50. Lipoprotein (a):

A. has structural similarities to fibrinogen
B. is produced in the liver
C. is an independent risk factor for ischaemic heart disease
D. tends to be higher in whites than blacks
E. is not affected by hormone replacement therapy

51. After the menopause:

A. rapid acceleration in bone loss tends to occur after about fifteen years from the last menstrual period
B. the commonest cause of death is myocardial infarction
C. if hormone replacement therapy is prescribed, a progestagen must always be given in conjunction with an oestrogen
D. the minimum dose of conjugated oestrogen which is needed to protect against bone loss is 0.625 mg daily
E. hormone replacement therapy should not be given if the woman has hypercholesterolaemia

52. Rabies:

A. is most prevalent in foxes in Europe
B. can only be contracted by biting (or licking)
C. can be vaccinated against after exposure
D. is usually fatal after clinical features appear
E. is best diagnosed by the corneal smear test

53. Glucose-6-phosphate dehydrogenase deficiency (G6PD):

A. causes a defect in the Embden–Meyerhof pathway
B. has an autosomal recessive inheritance
C. can be precipitated by nitrofurantoin
D. is a recognised cause of haemolytic anaemia
E. can be precipitated by eating peas

54. The following are risks for the development of schizophrenia:

A. maternal influenza in mid-pregnancy
B. living near high power cables
C. latitude of place of birth
D. family history
E. obstetric complications

55. Regarding diabetic retinopathy:

A. most patients with insulin-dependent diabetes will have evidence of retinopathy after 20 years of the disease
B. it tends to improve during pregnancy
C. intraretinal microvascular abnormalities are consistent with pre-proliferative changes
D. when proliferative retinopathy is diagnosed it is desirable to improve glycaemic control as quickly as possible to reduce chances of haemorrhage
E. a deterioration in visual acuity when using a pinhole is consistent with the presence of macular oedema

56. Obstructive sleep apnoea:

A. is a technical term for snoring
B. affects adults only
C. is due to episodic pharyngeal collapse
D. is a recognised risk factor for ischaemic heart disease
E. may be treated with acetazolamide

57. **In cardiopulmonary resuscitation:**

A.   age is a predictor of outcome
B.   approximately 50% of survivors can expect to leave hospital
C.   DC cardioversion should not be attempted if the patient is not connected to a cardiac monitor
D.   it is equally satisfactory to give adrenaline down the endotracheal tube or by peripheral vein
E.   a satisfactory neurological outcome cannot be obtained if anoxia has been present for more than 10 minutes

58. *Helicobacter pylori:*

A.   infection causing gastritis is often associated with histologically normal mucosa
B.   infection can be detected by ^{12}C-urease breath test
C.   antibodies are present in the serum of most patients with *Helicobacter pylori*-associated gastritis
D.   can be eradicated by a combination of H_2 antagonists and antibiotics
E.   is a rare cause of haemorrhagic colitis

59. *Herpes simplex* **encephalitis:**

A.   is more common in women
B.   may be preceded by gustatory hallucinations
C.   can present with an ascending paralysis
D.   is made less probable by an EEG finding of slow-wave abnormality
E.   if treated is usually associated with a complete recovery

17

60. Primary hyperparathyroidism:

A. may be caused by carcinoma of the parathyroid glands
B. is rarely asymptomatic
C. should be treated with low calcium diets if parathyroidectomy is not carried out
D. should be treated by parathyroidectomy if hypertension is present
E. in patients over 70 years of age should be treated surgically

Answers

1.   A – T; B – F; C – T; D – T; E – F

Outcome is not improved by giving steroids in haemorrhagic or infarct-associated cerebral oedema [1]. Studies using serial CT scans have shown spontaneous haemorrhagic transformation to occur in up to 40% of patients with cardioembolic stroke [2]. Because cerebral autoregulation is impaired in the acute phase of a stroke, lowering of blood pressure by hypotensive agents may worsen the patient's condition by reducing cerebral blood flow still further.

1.   Oppenheimer S, Hachinski V. Complications of acute stroke. Lancet. 1992;339:721–4.
2.   Hart RG. Cardiogenic embolism to the brain. Lancet. 1992;339:589–94.

2.   A – F; B – F; C – T; D – F; E – F

Acute pancreatitis is idiopathic in 10–30% of cases [1]. It may be a side-effect of sodium valproate therapy. When secondary to alcohol, it has an overall mortality of about 5% compared with 10–25% for gallstone-associated and idiopathic pancreatitis [2]. *Chronic* pancreatitis is associated with pancreatic cancer, especially the tropical and hereditary forms of the disease [3].

1.   Steinberg WM. Acute pancreatitis – never leave a stone unturned. N Engl J Med. 1992;326:635–7.
2.   Trapnell JE, Duncan EHL. Patterns of incidence in acute pancreatitis. Br Med J. 1975;2:179–83.
3.   Warshaw AL, Fernández-del Castillo C. Pancreatic carcinoma. N Engl J Med. 1992;326:455–65.

3.   A – T; B – T; C – T; D – T; E – T

Amiodarone and sulphasalazine cause interstitial lung disease, nebulised pentamidine is linked with pneumothorax, aspirin can cause bronchospasm and the contraceptive pill predisposes to pulmonary embolus.

Rosenow EC et al. Drug induced pulmonary disease. Chest. 1992;102:239–50.

4.   A – T; B – F; C – F; D – F; E – F

Approximately 80% of patients with lupus anticoagulant have ELISA antiphospholipid antibody, but only 10–50% of patients with antiphospholipid antibody have lupus anticoagulant [1]. Recent development of SLE with rapidly progressive renal failure is associated with a more favourable prognosis than the slowly progressive severe disease [2]. Plasmapheresis is not helpful in the treatment of severe lupus nephritis [3,4].

1.   Lockshin MD. Antiphospholipid antibody syndrome. JAMA. 1992;268:1451–3.
2.   Cheigh JS, Stenzel KH. End-stage renal disease in systemic lupus erythematosis. Am J Kid Dis. 1993;21:2–8.
3.   Glassock RJ. Intensive plasma exchange in crescentic glomerulonephritis: help or no help? Am J Kid Dis. 1992;20:270–5.
4.   Lewis EJ et al. A controlled trial of plasmapheresis therapy in severe lupus nephritis. N Engl J Med. 1992;326:1373–9.

5.   A – T; B – F; C – T; D – F; E – T

Poor glycaemic control in non-insulin-dependent diabetes is associated with elevation in plasma triglycerides and reduction in HDL [1]. Changes in total cholesterol and LDL are inconsistent. Well-controlled IDDM patients have normal or elevated HDL. Anion-exchange resins tend to increase triglycerides and are therefore not appropriate for the treatment of mixed hyperlipidaemia. Nephrotic syndrome secondary to any cause is associated with elevated cholesterol and triglycerides.

1.   Betteridge DJ. Lipids, diabetes and vascular disease: the time to act. Diab Med. 1989;6:195–218.

6.   A – F; B – F; C – T; D – F; E – F

The main site of absorption is the proximal small intestine, and is by an active transport mechanism utilising either transferrin or mobilferrin. Free iron is very toxic and it is therefore always bound to ferritin or transferrin. Inhibition of absorption occurs due to anything which firstly speeds up intestinal transit or secondly lowers pH. Fibre, tea, coffee and phosphates inhibit absorption. Total stores are 3–5 g, each pregnancy 'costs' 500–1000 mg, a menstrual period 20 mg and the usual daily turnover is about 1 mg. The main storage site is the reticuloendothelial system.

Massey MC. Microcytic anaemia. Med Clin N Am. 1992;76(3):549–66.

7. A – F; B – T; C – T; D – T; E – F

Cytokines are mediators of the inflammatory response and are produced by macrophages, lymphocytes and some other cells. They stimulate synthesis of acute phase proteins and 'switch on' fibroblasts and synthetic cells (GM CSF, for example, is a cytokine). Endotoxin is the cell wall constituent of Gram-negative bacteria which initiates septic shock, principally via tumour necrosis factor (which is a cytokine).

Woo P. The central role of cytokines in inflammation. In: Seymour CA (ed). Horizons in medicine, No. 3. Royal College of Physicians, London. 1991:223–30.

8. A – T; B – T; C – F; D – T; E – F

Mitral valve prolapse prevalence rates are 4–17% in women and 2–12% in men. Prevalence falls with increasing age in women, but remains static in men. Most people have no symptoms, but 60% of people with non-specific symptoms and the condition ('mitral valve prolase syndrome') have chest pain. Infective endocarditis occurs in 2–8% of patients with mitral valve prolapse, and postmortems have shown thrombi on mitral valve leaflets in patients who have died of cerebral emboli. The commonest indication for mitral valve replacement in elderly people is myxomatous degeneration and mitral valve prolapse.

Alpert MA. Mitral valve prolapse. Br Med J. 1993;306:943–4.

9. A – F; B – T; C – T; D – T; E – T

Seminomas account for 50% of testicular germ cell tumours [1]. About 80% of patients with testicular teratoma will have elevated α-FP, hCG or both. Metastatic bone involvement may lead to bone pain. Mediastinal germ cell tumours may occur in association with Klinefelter's syndrome and acute myeloid leukaemia.

1. Mead GM. Testicular cancer and related neoplasms. Br Med J. 1992;304:1426–9.

10. A – F; B – T; C – T; D – F; E – T

Phenothiazines, butyrophenones, and thioxanthines can all cause NMS. It is often associated with elevated creatine kinase levels. Treatment includes general supportive measures, rehydration, discontinuation of the offending drug, and administration of a central dopamine agonist or peripheral muscle relaxant (e.g. dantrolene).

1. Nierenberg D et al. Facilitating prompt diagnosis and treatment of the neuroleptic malignant syndrome. Clin Pharmacol Ther. 1991;50:580–6.

11. A – T; B – F; C – T; D – T; E – T

Evans JG, Williams JF. Oxford textbook of geriatric medicine. Oxford Medical Publications, OUP, 1992.

12. A – F; B – T; C – F; D – F; E – T

Legionnaire's disease is notifiable in Northern Ireland and Scotland, but in England and Wales infections are monitored by voluntary reporting to the Communicable Disease Surveillance Centre. Most cases occur in people between the ages of 40 and 70 years with males affected three times more commonly than females. Most cases are sporadic, with less than 25% occurring in outbreaks. Pontiac fever is also caused by a *Legionella* organism, but no fatalities have been recorded.

Joint Health and Safety Executive Department of Health Working Group on Legionellosis. The prevention and control of Legionellosis: review and forward look. Health and Safety Executive and the Department of Health, 1992.

13. A – F; B – T; C – T; D – F; E – T

The classical colour changes in Raynaud's phenomenon are white, blue, and then red [1]. It may be associated with a number of conditions (e.g. connective tissue disorders, cervical rib, cryoglobulinaemia) and may be provoked by exposure to vinyl chloride. Cervical sympathectomy is associated with a high relapse rate of Raynaud's.

1. Belch JJF. Management of Raynaud's phenomenon. Hospital Update. 1990;16:391–2, 395–6, 398–400.

14. A – T; B – F; C – F; D – F; E – F

Hyperosmolar non-ketotic coma (HONK) may be the presenting feature of diabetes, especially in the elderly. Compared with ketoacidosis (DKA), fluid replacement should be more cautious but insulin doses need to be lower because patients are more insulin sensitive. Cerebral oedema is not usually a feature of HONK but may occur during the treatment of DKA [1–2]. HONK has a worse prognosis than DKA (40% vs 10%). Patients generally do not require insulin in the long term after the successful treatment of HONK.

1. Hammond P, Wallis S. Cerebral oedema in diabetic ketoacidosis. Br Med J. 1992;305:203–4.
2. Hamblin PS et al. Deaths associated with diabetic ketoacidosis and hyperosmolar coma 1973–1988. Med J Aust. 1989;151(8):439, 441–2, 444.

15. A – F; B – T; C – T; D – F; E – T

70% of PO_4 is absorbed in the proximal small intestine. There is an increase in calcitriol with falling dietary PO_4, but, because of raised PTH, renal excretion is relatively spared. It is, however, important to treat hyperphosphataemia to try and reduce the magnitude of secondary hyperparathyroidism, especially in dialysis patients. Dairy products tend to contain a lot of PO_4.

Delmez JA, Slatopolsky E. Hyperphosphataemia: its consequences and treatment in patients with chronic renal disease. Am J Kidney Dis. 1992;XIX(4):303–16.

16. A – T; B – T; C – T; D – T; E – F

'Ecstasy' is a synthetic amphetamine derivative which has a wide range of adverse effects including anorexia, trismus, sweating, hypertension and hepatomegaly [1–2]. Acute severe complications include convulsions, DIC, hyperpyrexia, rhabdomyolysis and acute renal failure.

1. Henry JA. Ecstasy and the dance of death. Br Med J. 1992;305:5–6.
2. Henry JA et al. Toxicity and deaths from 3,4-methylenedioxymetamphetamine ('ecstasy'). Lancet. 1992;340:384–7.

17. A – F; B – T; C – T; D – T; E – F

Conduction delay tends to make the sound of valve closure (i.e. S1) quieter, and the converse is also true. Pericardial effusions make everything quieter!

Swanton RH. Cardiology. Blackwell Scientific Publications, London. 1989:13–4.

18. A – F; B – T; C – T; D – T; E – T

Radioimmunoassays which are commonly used measure total, rather than free, cortisol [1]. Enzyme inducers increase the clearance of dexamethasone and may therefore be associated with false positive results. More than 90% of patients with Cushing's syndrome fail to show a cortisol rise during an insulin tolerance test (provided adequate hypoglycaemia is attained), whilst depressed subjects show a normal rise. Ectopic CRH is a rare cause of Cushing's syndrome.

Trainer PJ, Grossman A. The diagnosis and differential diagnosis of Cushing's syndrome. Clin Endocrinol. 1991;34:317–30.

19. A – F; B – T; C – T; D – F; E – F

Retinal damage occurs somewhere between 97 and 105 minutes after central retinal artery occlusion, but some useful return of vision may occur up to 12 hours. The main causes are embolic (c. 50% cardiac association, including MVP), atheromatous occlusion in situ, inflammatory (e.g. giant cell arteritis), angiospasm (e.g. 'complicated' migraine) and hydrostatic arterial occlusion (either raised intra-occular pressure, i.e. glaucoma, or local/regional hypotension).

Wray SH. The management of acute visual failure. J Neurol Neurosurg Psych. 1993;56:234–40.

20. A – T; B – T; C – T; D – F; E – F

There are a large number of drugs which can cause constipation [1]. These include diuretics, vinca alkaloids, antiparkinsonian drugs, disopyramide, and cholestyramine. Cimetidine may cause diarrhoea.

1. Bateman DN. Management of constipation. Prescribers' J. 1991;31:7–15.

21. A – F; B – F; C – F; D – F; E – T

PCP can occur in any immunosuppressed patient, and human pneumocystitis has never been successfully cultured. The usual presentation is with malaise, breathlessness and a dry cough. The X-ray may be normal or show diffuse alveolar infiltrates, classically with sparing of the costophrenic angles. If the condition is of more than mild severity, steroids are shown to improve the outcome. Prophylaxis in HIV patients is indicated when the CD4 count is less than 200 cells/mm.

Masur H. Prevention and treatment of pneumocystis pneumonia. N Engl J Med. 1992;327(26):1853–60.

22. A – T; B – F; C – T; D – T; E – T

ANCA are a diverse group of antibodies, of all immunoglobulin classes, which enter granulocytes reacting either with perinuclear antigens (p-ANCA) or cytoplasmic elements (actually an enzyme, proteinase 3), c-ANCA. There are also atypical ANCAs. It is present in 5% of healthy people, 60–75% of patients with UC and is a sensitive and specific marker for Wegener's granulomatosis, as well as Churg–Strauss syndrome, PAN, RA, autoimmune liver disease and most vasculitides.

Kallenberg CGM et al. Antineutrophil cytoplasmic antibodies: A still-growing class of autoantibodies in inflammatory disorders. Am J Med. 1992;93:675–81.

23. A – T; B – T; C – F; D – F; E – T

Non-thyroidal illness can lead to alterations in the results of thyroid function tests for a number of reasons, including reduction in the peripheral conversion of T4 to T3, a decrease in thyroid hormone-binding proteins, and release of circulating inhibitors that prevent thyroid hormone binding [1]. Free T4 tends to fall during pregnancy, and TSH is the most reliable indicator of thyroid status in the second and third trimesters. (TSH is, however, sometimes low in the first trimester.) Although oestrogens increase TBG, free T4 remains normal because of a concomitant rise in total T4. No single biochemical test will reliably confirm thyroid dysfunction in patients on amiodarone, but it is possible for hyperthyroidism to be present when total T4 is within the normal range [2].

1. Felicetta JV. Effects of illness on thyroid function tests. Postgrad Med. 1989;85:213–20.
2. Kennedy RL et al. Amiodarone and the thyroid. Clin Chem. 1989;35:1882–7.

24. A – T; B – F; C – T; D – T; E – F

Acquired sideroblastic anaemia may be due to alcohol or other drugs such as isoniazid, cycloserine, and chloramphenicol [1]. Lead poisoning may also cause a sideroblastic anaemia as may malignant diseases of the bone marrow.

1. Bunch C. The blood in systemic disease. Med Int. 1991;96:3990–5.

25. A – T; B – F; C – F; D – T; E – F

The important thing to remember is that non-parametic tests are required where the distributions are not normal (Gaussian). There is often one statistics question in MRCP Part 1.

Swinscow TDV. Statistics at square one. British Medical Association, Tavistock Square, London. 1980.

26. A – T; B – T; C – F; D – F; E – F

Magnesium ions modulate calcium and potassium channels, as well as adenylate cyclase activity [1]. Magnesium competes with calcium to inhibit contractility of coronary arteries, as with other vascular smooth muscle. There are no absolute contraindications to iv magnesium therapy but the dose should be reduced in the presence of moderate to severe renal failure because of accumulation of magnesium. Short-term morbidity (in the form of incidence of left ventricular failure on the coronary care unit) and *mortality* have been found to be reduced when iv magnesium is used in the treatment of acute MI [2]. A meta-analysis has suggested that i.v. magnesium reduces the incidence of ventricular dysrhythmias in acute MI [3].

1. Woods KL. Possible pharmacological actions of magnesium in acute myocardial infarction. Br J Clin Pharmacol. 1991;32:3–10.
2. Woods KL et al. Intravenous magnesium sulphate in suspected acute myocardial infarction: results of the second Leicester Intravenous Magnesium Intervention Trial (LIMIT-2). Lancet. 1992;339:1553–8.
3. Horner SM et al. Efficacy of intravenous magnesium in acute myocardial infarction in reducing arrhythmias and mortality: meta-analysis of magnesium in acute myocardial infarction. Circulation. 1992;86:774–9.

27. A – F; B – F; C – F; D – T; E – T

Octreotide is a somatostatin analogue. It has no effect on ACTH production or posterior pituitary activity [1]. Its main indication is after pituitary surgery if growth hormone levels are still elevated [2]. It has been tried in a number of clinical settings, including the management of variceal bleeding, polycystic ovarian syndrome, gastroenteropancreatic tumours, psoriasis, and refractory diarrhoea associated with AIDS.

1. Editorial. All aboard for octreotide. Lancet. 1990;336:909–11.
2. Editorial. Octreotide steaming ahead. Lancet. 1992;339:837–9.

28. A – F; B – F; C – F; D – T; E – F

Symptoms usually appear when dopamine has fallen to only about 20% of normal due to various compensatory mechanisms. The tremor is 4–8 Hz, and 'pill-rolling'. Vertical gaze palsy suggests that the diagnosis is Steele–Richardson–Olszewski syndrome which responds poorly to therapy. Lewy bodies are also found in Alzheimer's disease, and healthy elderly people [1]. Selegiline has recently become a first-line treatment for *early* Parkinson's disease following the DATATOP study which suggested a possible disease-modifying role [2,3].

1. Playfer J. Parkinson's disease and other Parkinsonian syndromes. In: Tallis R (ed). The clinical neurology of old age. J Wiley & Sons, Chichester. 1989:127–40.
2. The Parkinson's study group. Effect of deprenyl on the progression of disability in early Parkinson's disease. N Engl J Med. 1989;321:1364–71.
3. The Parkinson's study group. Effects of tocopherol and deprenyl on the progression of disability in early Parkinson's disease. N Engl J Med. 1993;328:176–83.

29. A – T; B – T; C – F; D – T; E – F

Biliary output of cholesterol is increased and synthesis of bile acid is reduced by oestrogen therapy [1]. Gallstones are commoner in women than men across all age groups. About 80% of patients with gallbladder cancer have gallstones, with a particuarly high risk in those with longstanding stones or stones greater than 3 cm in diameter. Only radiolucent cholesterol stones can be dissolved with solvents such as methyl-tert-butyl ether [2].

1. Johnston DE, Kaplan MM. Pathogenesis and treatment of gallstones. N Engl J Med. 1993;328:412–21.
2. Sauerbruch T, Paumgartner G. Gallbladder stones: management. Lancet. 1991;338:1121–4.

30. A – F; B – F; C – T; D – T; E – T

Brucellosis is a zoonosis which, classically, is transmitted by the consumption of contaminated lamb, beef, or the milk of these animals: sheep don't bite! A live attenuated vaccine is used in cattle and this can cause infection in humans. The most serious manifestations are (aortic valve) endocarditis, meningo-encephalitis and visceral abscesses. Brucellosis is endemic in Spain.

Friedland JS. Uncommon infections: 7. Brucellosis. Prescriber's J. 1993;33(1):24–8.

31. A – T; B – T; C – T; D – T; E – T

Onset of gout before the age of 30 in men and in any premenopausal woman should raise the question of a specific enzyme defect leading to marked purine overproduction or an inherited defect in renal tubular handling [1]. Allopurinol can cause rashes, vasculitis, hepatitis, interstitial nephritis, and toxic epidermal necrolysis [2].

1. Dieppe PA. Investigation and management of gout in the young and elderly. Ann Rheum Dis. 1991;50:263–6.
2. Singh JZ, Wallace SL. The allopurinol hypersensitivity problem. Arthritis Rheum. 1986;29:82–9.

32. A – T; B – T; C – F; D – F; E – T

Human insulin is absorbed slightly more quickly than porcine insulin when given subcutaneously [1]. In a meta-analysis of combination sulphonylurea and insulin therapy in non-insulin-dependent diabetic (NIDD) patients, combination treatment was associated with a modest improvement in glycaemic control [2]. Metformin and insulin may be used in the treatment of the obese NIDD patient. There is no good evidence to support the notion that human insulin causes greater loss of warning symptoms compared with animal insulins in double-blind randomised crossover studies [3–5]. Patients who are most at risk of having recurrent severe hypoglycaemia are those on intensified insulin therapy and/or who have a past history of severe hypoglycaemia.

1. MacPherson JN, Feely J. Insulin. Br Med J. 1990;300:731–6.
2. Pugh JA et al. Is combination sulfonylurea and insulin therapy useful in NIDDM patients? A metaanalysis. Diabetes Care. 1992;15(8):953–9.
3. Gerich JE. Unawareness of hypoglycaemia and human insulin. Br Med J. 1992;305:324–5.
4. Colagiuri S et al. Double-blind crossover comparison of human and porcine insulins in patients reporting lack of hypoglycaemia awareness. Lancet. 1992;339:1432–5.
5. Maran A et al. Double-blind clinical and laboratory study of hypoglycaemia with human and porcine insulin in diabetic patients reporting hypoglycaemia unawareness after transferring to human insulin. Br Med J. 1993;306:167–71.

33. A – F; B – F; C – F; D – T; E – F

Microalbuminuria is defined as urinary excretion of albumin that is persistently elevated above normal which is not detectable by conventional semiquantitative test strips. It is only deemed present after infection and structural abnormalities of the urinary tract have been excluded [1]. It predicts mortality from cardiovascular disease in diabetic and elderly subjects. Most insulin-dependent diabetic patients with microalbuminuria have retinopathy, but usually this is of the background variety [2]. In microalbuminuric patients, strict metabolic control by continuous subcutaneous insulin infusion has been effective in reducing the albumin excretion rate [3–4]. Persistent elevation in albumin excretion rates is exceptional in the first five years of insulin-dependent diabetes.

1. Wincour PH. Microalbuminuria. Br Med J. 1992;304:1196–7.
2. Parving H-H et al. Prevalence of microalbuminuria, arterial hypertension, retinopathy and neuropathy in patients with insulin-dependent diabetes. Br Med J. 1988;296:156–60.
3. Bending JJ et al. Eight-month correction of hyperglycaemia in IDDM is associated with a significant and sustained reduction of urinary albumin excretion rates in patients with microalbuminuria. Diabetes. 1985;34(suppl 3):69–73.
4. Kroc Collaborative Study Group. Blood glucose control and the evolution of diabetic retinopathy and albuminuria: a preliminary multicenter trial. N Engl J Med. 1984;311:365–72.

34. A – T; B – T; C – T; D – T; E – T

Higgins EM, du Vivier AWP. Alcohol and the skin. Alcohol Alcoholism. 1992;27(6):595–602.

35. A – F; B – F; C – F; D – T; E – F

Balloon valvuloplasty is more likely to be successful in the long term if the valve cusps are pliable and not heavily calcified [1]. The combination of hydralazine and isosorbide dinitrate has been shown to reduce mortality compared with placebo [2]. Metolazone is a thiazide-like diuretic. Long-term digoxin therapy has been shown to improve symptoms and exercise tolerance in patients in sinus rhythm, but its effect on survival is unknown [3–5].

1. Hall R, Kirk R. Balloon dilatation of heart valves. Br Med J. 1992;305:487–8.
2. Conn JN et al. Effect of vasodilator therapy on mortality in chronic congestive cardiac failure. Results of a Veterans Administration cooperative study. N Engl J Med. 1986;314:1547–52.
3. Packer M. Treatment of chronic heart failure. Lancet. 1992;340:92–5.
4. DiBianco R et al. A comparison of oral milrinone, digoxin and their combination in the treatment of patients with chronic heart failure. N Engl J Med. 1989;320:677–83.
5. Packer M et al. Randomized, double-blind, placebo-controlled, withdrawal study of digoxin in patients with chronic heart failure treated with converting-enzyme inhibitors. J Am Coll Cardiol. 1992;19:260A.

36. A – T; B – F; C – F; D – F; E – T

Hyperprolactinaemia is a cause of both primary and secondary amenorrhoea – up to 20% of women with the latter have hyperprolactinaemia. Hyperprolactinaemia may be caused by *hypo*thyroidism. Prolactin levels are of no prognostic significance in pregnant women with prolactinomas: tumour expansion may occur without concomitant rise in prolactin [1]. Dopamine agonist therapy is often effective in rapidly reducing the effect of pressure of a macroadenoma upon surrounding structures [2]. The recurrence rate of prolactinoma after neurosurgery for a macroadenoma is high, as is the occurrence of hypopituitarism.

1. Molitch ME. Pregnancy and the hyperprolactinaemic woman. N Engl J Med. 1985;34:231–5.
2. Cunnah D, Besser M. Management of prolactinomas. Clin Endocrin. 1991;34:231–5.

37. A – T; B – T; C – F; D – T; E – F

Most 5HT receptors are in the brain except for $5HT_2$ (lung, platelets, arteries and gut) and $5HT_{1D}$ (carotid arterial tree). The latter are stimulated by sumitriptan causing vasodilatation and relief of migraine. Ecstasy causes 5HT release, while the new generation antiemetics (e.g. ondansetron) work by blocking $5HT_3$ receptors. Levels are low in depression although whether this is causal is not known.

Anon. Drugs affecting 5HT function. Drug Ther Bull. 1993;31(7):25–7.

38. A – F; B – T; C – T; D – T; E – F

Alcoholic cirrhosis is increasing, particularly in women. Binge drinkers 'rest' their liver, and have a better diet, and therefore a better outcome. Biopsy appearances can be variable, but some drugs can give a similar appearance. Renal tubular defects would suggest that the cause of cirrhosis is Wilson's disease, though alcoholics can get glomerular defects.

Sherlock S. Alcoholic liver disease. In: Salmon PR (ed). Key developments in gastroenterology. Wiley Medical, London. 1988:47–66.

39. A – T; B – F; C – F; D – F; E – T

Both A and B are characteristic pathological findings, the latter being associated with a worse outlook. Markers of RV failure, such as high RA pressure, are prognostic indicators: as the RV fails the output falls and the PA pressure then falls. Heart/lung transplant is the only proven treatment but drugs like nifedipine are thought to be helpful.

Uren NG, Oakley CM. The treatment of primary pulmonary hypertension. Br Heart J. 1991;66:119–21.

40. A – T; B – T; C – F; D – T; E – F

Urticarial vasculitis occurs in a number of connective tissue disorders of which SLE is the commonest [1]. It may occur in conjunction with angioedema/abdominal pain and arthralgias unrelated to a defined connective tissue disorder – this is known as the 'AHA syndrome': arthralgias/arthritis (A), hives (H), angio-oedema (A). Symptoms may be precipitated by alcohol, stress and exercise. Serum complement is either low or normal. Treatment is difficult and rarely is there response to antihistamines alone. Immunosuppressive therapy, antimalarials, and monoclonal antibodies directed against CD4 cells have been tried.

1. Asherson RA, Sontheimer R. Urticarial vasculitis and syndromes in association with connective tissue diseases. Ann Rheum Dis. 1991;50:743–4.

41. A – F; B – F; C – T; D – T; E – T

Phaeochromocytoma is a rare cause of hypertension with an incidence of 1 to 2 per 100 000 adults per year [1]. Malignancy occurs in about 10% of patients. Acute LVF is a recognised presentation of phaeochromocytoma [2]. MIBG is taken up by chromaffin cells and is used to locate the tumour. It has also been used in large doses to treat metastatic phaeochromocytoma. Patients with tumours which secrete adrenaline predominantly may present with hypotension rather than hypertension [3].

1. Sheps SG et al. Recent developments in the diagnosis and treatment of phaeochromocytoma. Mayo Clin Proc. 1990;65:88–95.
2. Editorial. Phaeochromocytoma still surprises. Lancet. 1990;335:1189–90.
3. Ross EJ, Griffith DNW. The clinical presentation of phaeochromocytoma. Q J Med. 1989;266:485–96.

42. A – F; B – T; C – F; D – F; E – T

ITP is due to a platelet-specific IgG, which can cross the placenta, causing platelet destruction, with consequent increased synthesis. Splenectomy is an effective treatment in 80% of cases, but, because of the long-term post-splenectomy risks, is normally resorted to only after trial of steroids and i.v. immunoglobulin.

Provan AB. Management of adult idiopathic thrombocytopenic purpura. Prescriber's J. 1992;32(5):193–200.

43. A – F; B – T; C – T; D – F; E – F

About 10% of drowning is 'dry' drowning in which water is not aspirated into the lungs. It is important to distinguish between sea and fresh water drowning: fresh water destabilises surfactant causing alveolar collapse, unlike seawater. Sea drowners are intravascularly dry, because of osmotic flow into the lungs; the reverse happens in fresh water. CPAP is valuable in both types of drowning, but no convincing value has been shown for steroids.

Modell JH. Drowning. N Engl J Med. 1993;328(4):253–6.

44. A – T; B – F; C – F; D – T; E – T

Narcolepsy is an unusual condition with an HLA linkage that is
98–100%, and is characterised by a clinical triad of daytime sleepiness,
sleep paralysis and cataplexy. The latter symptom occurs in virtually no
other condition. Amphetamines are the classical treatment but some
success has been claimed for selegiline and tricyclics.

Aldrich MS. Narcolepsy. N Engl J Med. 1990;323:389–94.

45. A – T; B – T; C – T; D – T; E – F

Airport malaria has been reported in the UK and Switzerland. Babies
with malaria have also been born in the USA to pregnant immigrant
women, implying congenital transmission. Intravenous quinine is the
drug of choice in severe malaria, but the anti-arrhythmic quinidine may
also be used. Although *P. falciparum* is only in the peripheral blood for
18–24 hours of its 48-hour lifecycle, causing some negative smears, in
general terms the prognosis is proportional to the % parasitaemia;
>5% constitutes severe disease.

Hoffman SL. Diagnosis, treatment and prevention of malaria. Med Clin N Am.
1992;76(6):1327–55.

46. A – F; B – F; C – T; D – T; E – T

Behçet's disease is an illness of the second to fourth decade [1]. Renal
impairment is uncommon but when it occurs is often due to
amyloidosis. Vasculitis of the coronary arteries may lead to myocardial
infarction. Thalidomide is effective in the treatment of severe recurrent
aphthous stomatitis; cyclosporin is more effective in the treatment of
ocular problems and mucocutaneous lesions.

1.   Wechsler B, Piette JC. Behçet's disease. Br Med J. 1992;304:1199–1200.

47. A – T; B – F; C – F; D – T; E – T

C-peptide levels increase in parallel with plasma insulin in patients with insulinoma, but proinsulin is markedly increased because of a defect in the conversion of proinsulin to insulin [1,2]. Factitious hypoglycaemia due to sulphonylurea ingestion is confirmed by detecting the drug and/or its metabolites in plasma or urine. C-peptide is markedly elevated, and proinsulin only mildly increased in such cases. Fasting hypoglycaemia due to antiinsulin antibodies may occur in SLE, Graves' disease, rheumatoid arthritis, multiple myeloma and benign monoclonal gammopathy.

1. Polonsky KS. A practical approach to fasting hypoglycaemia. N Engl J Med. 1992;326:1020–1.
2. Marks V, Teale JD. Tumours producing hypoglycaemia. Diabetes Metab Rev. 1991;7:79–91.

48. A – F; B – F; C – T; D – F; E – F

Isotope renography will, at best, detect 90% of renal artery stenoses [1,2]. There is a high prevalence of atherosclerotic renal artery stenosis in the elderly population 3. and up to 40% of these subjects will have renal impairment. Diuretics are thought not to be helpful in the treatment of renovascular hypertension because blood pressure is inversely related to the total exchangeable sodium concentration.

1. Carmichael DJS et al. Detection and investigation of renal artery stenosis. Lancet. 1986;327:667–70.
2. Davidson RA, Wilcox CS. Newer tests for the diagnosis of renovascular hypertension. JAMA. 1992;268:3353–8.
3. Scoble JE, Hamilton G. Atherosclerotic renovascular disease. Br Med J. 1990;300:1670–1.

49. A – T; B – T; C – F; D – T; E – T

Initially cerebral blood flow is increased to cope with the increased metabolism. Later cardiovascular compromise supervenes with associated multiorgan failure and loss of movements. The cerebral circulation is particularly vulnerable because of raised ICP. Ninety minutes is the absolute maximum time allowed to obtain seizure control by medical means.

Shorvon S. Tonic clonic status epilepticus. J Neurol Neurosurg Psych. 1993;56:125–34.

50. A – F; B – T; C – T; D – F; E – F

Lp (a) contains one (or two) molecules of apo (a) linked to apo B100 by a disulphide bridge [1]. Apo (a) is related to plasminogen. Lp (a) concentrations tend to be higher in blacks, where this is not associated with an increase in ischaemic heart disease, in contrast to an increased risk in whites. Oestrogens do not seem to affect Lp (a) levels, but norethisterone has been shown to reduce Lp (a) in postmenopausal women [2].

1. Scott J. Lipoprotein (a). Br Med J. 1991;303:663–4.
2. Rosengren A et al. Lipoprotein (a) concentrations in postmenopausal women taking norethisterone. Br Med J. 1991;303:694.

51. A – F; B – T; C – F; D – T; E – F

Most bone is lost during the first 3–6 years after the menopause. A progestagen is not necessary as part of HRT in women without a uterus. Minimum daily doses to prevent bone loss are 0.625 mg of conjugated oestrogen, 15 µg of ethinyl oestradiol, and 50 µg of transdermal oestradiol. Natural oestrogens cause a reduction in total and LDL cholesterol, and an elevation in HDL; they have no effect on triglycerides.

1. Riggs BL, Melton III LJ. The prevention and treatment of osteoporosis. N Engl J Med. 1992;327:620–7.
2. Jacobs HS, Loeffler FE. Postmenopausal hormone replacement therapy. Br Med J. 1992;305:1403–8.

52. A – T; B – F; C – T; D – F; E – F

Rabies may also be contracted by inhalation (in bat-infested caves) and iatrogenically by transplant in corneal grafting. The main European reservoir is foxes, but this varies around the world with bats, mongeese, and other canine animals also important. There are 3 recorded cases of survival from clinical rabies, but admittedly this is the exception rather than the rule. Diagnosis is either from the biting animal or by skin biopsy or, in the unvaccinated patient, by antibody titre.

Warrell MJ, Warrell DA. Rabies. Med Int. 1992;106:4440–6.

53.   A – F; B – F; C – T; D – T; E – F

G6PD is the most common defect of the hexose-monophosphate shunt (the most common abnormality of the Embden Meyerhof pathway is pyruvate kinase deficiency). Inheritance is X-linked. Because the RBCs are unable to generate enough glutathione, they are susceptible to oxidation (e.g. by drugs, uremia, acidosis and fava beans).

Tabbara IA. Haemolytic anaemias. Med Clin N Am. 1992;76(3):649–68.

54.   A – T; B – F; C – F; D – T; E – T

Perinatal and prenatal influences are increasingly recognised as risks for schizophrenia. Latitude of place of birth is true of multiple sclerosis. The concordance rate for MZ twins is 40–50%, indicating a genetic contribution of about 75%.

Waddington JL. Schizophrenia: developmental neuroscience and pathobiology. Lancet. 1993;341:531–5.

55.   A – T; B – F; C – T; D – F; E – T

90% of diabetic patients will have retinopathy after 20 years of disease duration [1]. Retinopathy tends to deteriorate during pregnancy [2]. Pre-proliferative changes include cotton wool spots, multiple large blot haemorrhages, intraretinal microvascular abnormalities, venous bleeding, loops, and reduplication, and arterial sheathing. Several prospective studies [3–5] have shown a temporary deterioration in retinopathy (lasting up to one year) in patients who improve their glycaemic control acutely. In the long term, good diabetic control is associated with an improvement in retinopathy.

1. Krowlewski AS et al. Risk of proliferative diabetic retinopathy in juvenile-onset type 1 diabetes: a 40 year follow-up study. Diabetes Care. 1986;9:443–52.
2. Klein BEK et al. Effect of pregnancy on progression of diabetic retinopathy. Diabetes Care. 1990;13:34–40
3. Lauritzen T et al. (Steno Study Group). Two-year experience with continuous subcutaneous insulin infusion in relation to retinopathy and neuropathy. Diabetes. 1985;34 suppl (3):74–9.
4. Kroc Collaborative Study Group. Blood glucose control and the evolution of diabetic retinopathy and albuminuria: a preliminary multicenter trial. N Engl J Med. 1984;311:365–72.
5. Dahl-Jorgensen et al. Rapid tightening of blood glucose control leads to transient deterioration of retinopathy in insulin-dependent diabetes mellitus: the Oslo study. Br Med J. 1986;293:1195–9.

56. A – F; B – F; C – T; D – T; E – F

As the name implies obstructive sleep apnoea (OSA) is due to frequent (>10/h) episodes of pharyngeal collapse, to which a variety of factors predispose. It occurs in children (usually due to tonsils), and can lead to systemic and pulmonary hypertension, and IHD. Acetazolamide causes a metabolic acidosis and is therefore sometimes useful in central sleep apnoea, but not OSA.

Nasser S, Rees PJ. Sleep apnoea: causes, consequences and treatment. Br J Clin Prac. 1992;46(1):39–43.

57. A – F; B – F; C – F; D – F; E – F

Poor predictors of outcome include a previously housebound lifestyle, cancer, renal failure, and pneumonia, but not age. The best ever results showed a 14% discharge rate (from the Beth Israel Hospital in Boston) [1]. If a monitor is not available, a 200J DC shock should be applied, as VF is much the most treatable rhythm. Recent studies have shown that ETT adrenaline is not absorbed [2]. Famous cases exist of children being resuscitated after falling into frozen lakes after long periods, but the discharge rate for patients brought to A&E with no pulse was 1 in 211 in a recent study [3].

1. Bedell SE et al. Survival after cardiopulmonary resuscitation in the hospital. N Engl J Med. 1983;309(10):569–76.
2. Niemann JT. Cardiopulmonary resuscitation. N Engl J Med. 1992;327(15):1075–80.
3. Lewis LM et al. Is emergency department resuscitation of out of hospital cardiac arrest victims who arrive pulseless worthwhile? Am J Emerg Med. 1990;8(2):118–20.

58. A – F; B – F; C – T; D – T; E – F

The presence of histologically normal mucosa virtually excludes *H. pylori* infection [1]. The urease breath test uses ^{13}C as the tracer. IgG antibodies to *H. pylori* are present in most patients with infection, but IgA and/or IgM may also be present [2]. Both H_2 antagonists and proton-pump inhibitors (when used in combination with antibiotics) have been shown to eradicate the organism [3,4].

1. Graham DY. Treatment of peptic ulcers caused by Helicobacter pylori. N Engl J Med. 1993;328:349–50.
2. Kosunen TU et al. Diagnostic value of decreasing IgG, IgA and IgM antibody titres after eradication of Helicobacter pylori. Lancet. 1992;339:893–5.
3. Hentschel E et al. Effect of ranitidine and amoxycillin and metronidazole on the eradication of Helicobacter pylori and the recurrence of duodenal ulcer. N Engl J Med. 1993;328:308–12.
4. Bayerdorffer E et al. High dose omeprazole treatment combined with amoxycillin eradicates Helicobacter pylori. Gastroenterology. 1992;102:A38.

59. A – F; B – T; C – F; D – F; E – F

The virus has a predilection for the temporal lobes (hence B, giving the characteristic EEG finding of temporal lobe slowing. Rabies and EBV can cause an ascending paralysis, but not HSV. There is no gender preponderance. Mortality, used to be c.70%, reduced to a morbidity of about 40% in the acyclovir era.

Bale JF. Viral encephalitis. Med Clin N Am. 1993;77(1):25–42

60. A – T; B – F; C – F; D – F; E – F

Primary hyperparathyroidism is usually due to a single benign adenoma, but may be due to multiple adenomas, parathyroid hyperplasia or carcinoma of the parathyroid [1]. It commonly is discovered as an incidental finding on biochemical testing. There is no place for the use of low calcium diets in this condition. Parathyroidectomy rarely cures sustained hypertension which may be present prior to surgery. There is no evidence to support the possibility that parathyroidectomy in the elderly has a beneficial effect on long-term survival.

1. Davies M. Primary hyperparathyroidism: aggressive or conservative treatment? Clin Endocrinol. 1992;36:325–32.

Section 2 – General Medicine

1. **The following are true concerning pulmonary tuberculosis:**

A. one negative sputum smear is sufficient to demonstrate that a patient is not infectious

B. smear-positive patients need isolation until acid alcohol-fast bacilli are no longer visible in the sputum

C. it is not a notifiable disease

D. chemoprophylaxis should be given to all children (aged 0–5) of smear-positive adults

E. it affects 50% of AIDS patients in the UK

2. **Dermatomyositis and polymyositis:**

A. are more common in men than women

B. produce muscle weakness more commonly than muscle tenderness

C. both commonly produce arthralgia

D. when associated with interstitial lung disease is related to the presence of the anti-Jo-1 antibody

E. both show capillary damage on muscle histology

3. **The following are true of epilepsy:**

A. myoclonic seizure is an example of generalised epilepsy

B. rolling movements are more common in pseudoseizures compared with true epileptic attacks

C. the commonest cause of recent-onset epilepsy in elderly patients is a cerebral tumour

D. sodium valproate therapy during pregnancy is associated with an increased risk of spina bifida in the fetus

E. lamotrigine acts by inhibiting GABA transaminase

4. **The syndrome of inappropriate antidiuresis:**

A. is a recognised feature of cerebral abscess
B. is a recognised feature of pneumothorax
C. may occur in patients with increased thirst inappropriate to the level of hyponatraemia
D. is characterised by inappropriately high urinary osmolality relative to plasma osmolality, with reduced urinary sodium excretion
E. if treated with rapid administration of hypertonic saline may lead to quadraparesis

5. **The following statements regarding hepatitis C are correct:**

A. only 10% of infected patients develop cirrhosis
B. it is associated with hepatocellular carcinoma
C. it is associated with glomerulonephritis
D. it is more easily sexually transmissible than hepatitis B
E. treatment with α-interferon has been shown to be of benefit in chronic hepatitis C in randomised controlled trials

6. **Hair loss:**

A. may be a feature of psoriasis
B. may occur in the polycystic ovarian syndrome
C. occurring in the post-partum period usually resolves within three months
D. in alopecia areata has a poor prognosis for regrowth if the onset is in childhood
E. leading to baldness is common in eunuchs

7. **The following are correctly paired:**

A. tricuspid stenosis and prominent 'a' wave
B. atrial fibrillation and prominent 'a' wave
C. tamponade and loss of y descent
D. cannon 'a' waves and complete heart block
E. precipitous y descent and aortic stenosis

8. **In the nephrotic syndrome:**

A. both serum total cholesterol and triglycerides are usually elevated
B. serum HDL cholesterol tends to be reduced
C. occurring in a diabetic patient, diabetic nephropathy is rarely the underlying cause for the heavy proteinuria
D. patients should be encouraged to have a very high dietary protein intake in order to compensate for the marked proteinuria
E. renal vein thrombosis is a recognised complication

9. **Glibenclamide:**

A. is metabolised in the liver
B. has a longer half-life than chlorpropamide
C. is absorbed more effectively if given half an hour before, rather than with, a meal
D. may lead to death only if taken in overdose
E. is absolutely contraindicated in patients on β-blockers

10. **The following are true of leptospirosis:**

A. it causes a mild influenza-like illness in the majority of symptomatic patients
B. it may cause cholestatic jaundice
C. it may be complicated by myocarditis
D. treatment with penicillin may induce a transient exacerbation of symptoms with fever and hypotension
E. rats which harbour leptospira usually die within one month of excreting the organisms in the urine

11. In giant cell arteritis:

A.   the kidneys are often affected
B.   blindness may be due to central retinal artery occlusion
C.   patients may present in a non-specific manner with weight loss, general malaise and fever
D.   the erythrocyte sedimentation rate is greater than 100 mm/hour in about 95% of patients
E.   temporal artery biopsy is helpful in predicting the successful outcome of treatment withdrawal in patients treated with steroids

12. Lumbar puncture is always absolutely contraindicated if:

A.   there is raised intracranial pressure
B.   there is suspicion of thoracic cord compression
C.   there is skin sepsis at the entry site
D.   subarachnoid haemorrhage is suspected
E.   cerebellar signs are present

13. Growth hormone:

A.   is produced by basophilic cells of the anterior pituitary gland
B.   secretion throughout the day is pulsatile
C.   levels in malnutrition are low
D.   in excess produces carbohydrate intolerance
E.   secretion can be stimulated by L-dopa

14. The following are aetiological factors for fractured neck of femur:

A.   male sex
B.   previous oophorectomy
C.   excessive alcohol consumption
D.   postural hypotension
E.   peripheral neuropathy

15. **The following are valid indications for amniocentesis or chorionic villus sampling:**

A.   suspicion of Tay–Sachs disease
B.   maternal age over 30 years at time of delivery
C.   family history of cystic fibrosis
D.   maternal exposure to lithium
E.   paternal exposure to rubella

16. **Aortic dissection:**

A.   is categorised into two types by the DeBakey classification
B.   may present with paraplegia
C.   is always best treated surgically provided the anaesthetic risk is not too great
D.   can be evaluated by magnetic resonance imaging, which has a high sensitivity and specificity
E.   can be diagnosed by transoesophageal echocardiography, which has the additional advantage of being able to show the ostia and proximal coronary arteries

17. **In haemolytic anaemia:**

A.   the lifespan of a red cell is on average 150 days
B.   there is likely to be bilirubin in the urine
C.   if intravascular, there will be a reduced level of haptoglobins
D.   haemoglobinuria is a marker of severity
E.   *Mycoplasma* infection is a recognised cause

18. The following statements about diabetic neuropathy are correct:

A. improving glycaemic control does not alter the progression of peripheral neuropathy
B. amyotrophy rarely improves
C. when the oculomotor nerve is involved diplopia is characteristically of sudden onset
D. anticholinergic drugs may help in the treatment of gustatory sweating in autonomic neuropathy
E. ACE inhibitors may exacerbate diabetic impotence

19. In community-acquired pneumonias:

A. the commonest pathogen is *Mycoplasma pneumoniae*
B. erythromycin is the first-line antibiotic for psittacosis
C. the serum urea correlates with the severity of the illness
D. ciprofloxacin can be used as a single agent when the organism is not known
E. the pneumococcal antigen can be identified in the urine

20. In the treatment of osteoporosis:

A. oestrogens act directly on bone cells via high-affinity oestrogen receptors
B. intranasal calcitonin has been tried
C. biphosphonates act by inhibiting bone resorption
D. etridonate should only be given on an intermittent basis because long-term continuous treatment leads to impairment of newly synthesised bone matrix
E. sodium fluoride may produce a lower-extremity pain syndrome

21. Concerning anterior ischaemic optic neuropathy:

A. the optic nerve is supplied by a branch of the anterior cerebral artery
B. there is a recognised association with polyarteritis nodosa
C. an altitudinal field defect is unusual
D. the non-arteritic form is slowly progressive
E. most patients are more than 40 years old

22. Thyroid eye disease:

A. is a predictor of severity of thyroid disease
B. usually improves with treatment of the thyroid
C. risk is related to cigarette consumption
D. is linked to HLA DR4
E. is increasing in incidence

23. In irritable bowel syndrome:

A. women and men are affected equally
B. the symptoms can be produced by balloon distension of the rectum in a small number of patients
C. cisapride may accelerate colonic transit and may improve constipation
D. bloating can be exacerbated by fatty acids in some individuals
E. colonic transit times are longer in patients where diarrhoea predominates

24. The polymerase chain reaction (in vitro enzymatic DNA amplification):

A. can be used to amplify specimens several hundred years old
B. can be used to diagnose muscular dystrophy
C. can give false positive results even if the technique is correctly applied
D. is a good diagnostic test for malaria
E. requires a large specimen

25. Atrial fibrillation:

A. may be precipitated by acute hypovolaemia
B. which occurs paroxysmally is most effectively prevented by digoxin
C. of the 'lone' variety is associated with a particularly high risk of stroke
D. secondary to thyrotoxicosis is best controlled by β-blockers in the absence of heart failure
E. is associated with a high risk of stroke if there is a history of recent onset of congestive cardiac failure

26. In chronic renal failure:

A. serum erythropoietin is characteristically low when the anaemia is secondary to the renal impairment
B. the effects of erythropoietin are reduced in the presence of aluminium toxicity
C. human recombinant erythropoietin is recommended if the patient has angina which is aggravated by anaemia
D. secondary to polycystic kidney disease, hypertension is a late complication
E. the dose of atenolol generally needs to be reduced as the renal failure advances

27. In the management of acute severe hypercalcaemia:

A. correction of depleted intravascular volume by using isotonic saline will usually lower the serum calcium level by up to 0.6 mmol/L
B. calcitonin starts to lower serum calcium within a few hours after treatment is initiated
C. frusemide is helpful after rehydration has been achieved because of its effect on inhibition of calcium reabsorption in the descending limb of the loop of Henle
D. there is usually no place for emergency parathyroidectomy
E. corticosteroids are particularly effective if the hypercalcaemia is caused by primary hyperparathyroidism

28. Invasive aspergillosis:

A. is associated with a type III immune reaction
B. never occurs in immunocompetent individuals
C. is a common opportunistic infection in AIDS
D. can be treated with itraconazole
E. may be confirmed with an antigen test on serum

29. In rheumatoid arthritis:

A. histological study of human cartilage is normal
B. there is no evidence for a genetic susceptibility
C. IgM type autoantibodies may be demonstrated
D. non-steroidal anti-inflammatories are of no benefit
E. hydroxychloroquine is a recognised treatment

30. The following statements are true of headache:

A. cluster headache occurs more commonly in women
B. ptosis may occur during an attack of cluster headache
C. headache may be a presenting feature of sleep apnoea
D. migraine often deteriorates in pregnancy, especially in the third trimester
E. in the treatment of migraine, sumitriptan acts as a 5-HT agonist

31. **The following are true of impaired glucose tolerance (IGT):**

A. it is diagnosed by oral glucose tolerance test when the fasting venous plasma glucose is less than 6.7 mmol/L but rises to between 7.8 and 11.1 mmol/L two hours after a 75 g glucose load
B. people with IGT have a 20% annual risk of developing unequivocal diabetes
C. people with IGT have an increased cardiovascular morbidity compared with the normal population
D. 10% of those with IGT show evidence of diabetic retinopathy
E. as a group, people with IGT have hyperinsulinaemia when fasting and after a glucose load compared with the normal population

32. **The following are true of primary biliary cirrhosis:**

A. the clinical and biochemical state of the patient correlates well with the severity of histological changes in the liver
B. it is associated with Sjögren's syndrome
C. a rising bilirubin level is the most important indicator of a poor prognosis
D. ursodeoxycholic acid has been shown to improve biochemical abnormalities in primary biliary cirrhosis
E. it does not recur in patients treated with liver transplantation

33. **Antidotes exist to the following 'poisons':**

A. aspirin
B. atenolol
C. digoxin
D. nifedipine
E. chlorpromazine

34. Severe hypophosphataemia (serum phosphate of less than 0.32 mmol/L):

A. may occur in chronic alcoholism
B. is a feature of anorexia nervosa
C. may cause convulsions
D. may lead to respiratory failure due to diaphragmatic weakness
E. should generally be treated with intravenous phosphate if possible

35. Dexfenfluramine:

A. has stimulatory effects on the central nervous system when given in standard doses
B. has a known active metabolite
C. increases peripheral insulin sensitivity
D. may cause pulmonary hypertension
E. should not be given to patients on monoamine oxidase inhibitors

36. In asthma:

A. the neutrophil is the main mediator of the inflammatory response
B. there is a progressive decline in lung function, over a number of years
C. mortality is declining
D. reduction of inspiratory flow can be demonstrated on a flow-volume loop
E. inhaled steroids should be prescribed if more than occasional use of inhaled salbutamol is required

37. In the Guillain–Barré syndrome:

A. patients may present with footdrop
B. weakness may occur without any paraesthesia or sensory loss
C. nerve condition studies most commonly show evidence of demyelination
D. CSF protein is characteristically found to be greater than 2.5 g/L
E. pulsed intravenous methylprednisolone therapy has been shown to be as effective as plasma exchange in its treatment

38. Gynaecomastia:

A. may be caused by ketoconazole
B. may be caused by testicular tumours
C. which occurs in the neonatal period is due to transplacental passage of oestrogens
D. may be related to the presence of a prolactinoma
E. of the idiopathic variety is best treated by oral testosterone

39. Acyclovir:

A. inhibits the replication of herpes varicella-zoster virus
B. is a second-line treatment for active cytomegalovirus infection
C. should be given in reduced doses in patients with renal failure
D. crosses the placenta
E. prophylaxis of herpes simplex infections is beneficial in severely immunocompromised patients

40. When considering inserting a pacemaker in the elderly:

A. the commonest reason in patients over 70 years is AV conduction disorders
B. congestive cardiac failure rarely improves after pacing
C. digoxin should be ceased if the patient was previously taking it
D. 40% of patients with pacemakers will experience chronotropic incompetence
E. the commonest presenting symptom requiring pacing is syncope

41. The following features would suggest a primary rather than secondary cause for a patient's polycythaemia:

A. arterial oxygen saturation of 93%
B. platelet count of $350 \times 10^9/L$
C. normal leukocyte alkaline phosphatase score
D. splenomegaly
E. normal red cell mass

42. In diabetic ketoacidosis:

A. the serum sodium tends to be low at presentation
B. potassium should be added to the first bag of N/Saline given in the treatment because total body potassium is markedly reduced
C. serum phosphate may drop to potentially life-threatening levels during its treatment
D. bicarbonates should be given if arterial pH is less than 7.1
E. antibiotics should be prescribed routinely if the white cell count is elevated

43. Leprosy:

A. is not a notifiable disease
B. is transmitted via the female dustfly
C. is associated with a vigorous immune reaction in the lepromatous form
D. presents no risk to medical staff working in leprosy hospitals
E. cannot be cultured *in vitro*

44. In the transmissible spongiform encephalopathies:

A. Creutzfeldt–Jakob disease may show a dominant pattern of inheritance in 5–10% of cases
B. Kuru does not affect coordination
C. the pathology is different in humans and animals
D. the infectious agent has been identified
E. Creutzfeldt–Jakob disease can be transmitted to sheep

45. The polycystic ovarian syndrome:

A. is a rare cause of hirsutism
B. is characterised biochemically by elevated FSH:LH ratio, and serum testosterone
C. is associated with insulin resistance
D. may be associated with hyperprolactinaemia in up to 25% of cases
E. is best treated by using clomiphene

46. Ulcerative colitis:

A. may spare the rectum
B. presents most commonly in the over-40s
C. has a recognised association with fibrosing alveolitis
D. can be cured by proctocolectomy
E. should not be treated with sulphasalazine in women trying to start a family

47. Multiple myeloma:

A. is commoner in black people
B. when complicated by renal failure responds poorly to high fluid intake
C. when complicated by hyperviscosity syndrome may result in visual disturbance
D. has a worse prognosis in patients with a higher serum β_2-microglobulin level at diagnosis
E. when treated with combination chemotherapy has not been shown to be superior to intermittent melphalan in terms of survival

48. The diagnosis of cryptogenic organising pneumonitis (COP) is:

A. supported by the finding of patent alveolar ducts on lung biopsy
B. associated with rheumatoid arthritis
C. aided by bronchoalveolar lavage (BAL)
D. possible by serological tests
E. excluded if there is not a prompt response to steroids

49. The following are true of slow-acting antirheumatic drugs (SAARDs):

A. oral gold has been shown to be as effective as penicillamine and sulphasalazine
B. amongst the SAARDs, intramuscular gold is the most likely to be stopped because of toxicity
C. sulphasalazine may cause a leucopenia
D. thrombocytopenia associated with penicillamine therapy is an idiosyncratic side-effect
E. patients treated with methotrexate should be advised not to take concomitant cotrimoxazole therapy

50. Following trauma to the head the following may occur:

A. parasympathetically mediated rise in cardiac output
B. bradycardia
C. myocardial ischaemia
D. non-cardiac pulmonary oedema
E. increased oxygen consumption

51. Radioiodine:

A. is the treatment of choice for toxic multinodular goitre
B. is associated with hypothyroidism in up to 40% of patients 25 years after treatment
C. is associated with a small but significant increase in the incidence of leukaemia
D. is contraindicated if Graves ophthalmopathy is present
E. should be given whilst a thyrotoxic patient is on carbimazole to prevent early release of more thyroid hormone into the circulation

52. In Wilson's disease:

A. heterozygous phenotype should be treated
B. prognosis is unrelated to caeruloplasmin levels
C. hepatocellular carcinoma is a common event
D. renal tubular acidosis is a feature
E. urinary copper excretion is reduced

53. When ascending to high altitude (e.g. >3000 m):

A. there is increased urinary bicarbonate secretion
B. tachycardia resolves within 24 hours
C. pregnant women are at particular risk
D. the likelihood of cerebral oedema is unrelated to the speed of ascent
E. retinopathy is common

54. In hypertrophic obstructive cardiomyopathy (HOCM):

A. the ratio of septal to anterior left ventricular wall thickness on echocardiography must be at least 1:3
B. a rapid upstroke pulse is only found in about one-third of patients
C. there may be mutations in the myosin heavy chain in familial forms
D. there is no improvement in survival with amiodarone
E. the most useful predictor for sudden death is the echocardiographic appearance of the heart

55. Diabetic nephropathy:

A. often develops within 5 years of the onset of insulin-dependent DM
B. has a declining incidence 20 years after the onset of IDDM
C. may be predicted by the development of microalbuminuria
D. is associated with the same mortality as other causes of end-stage renal failure
E. may be retarded by appropriate antihypertensive therapy

56. *Giardia lamblia* infection:

A. is more common in homosexual men
B. is characterised by foul-smelling flatulence
C. is not a cause of malabsorbtion
D. may be more successfully diagnosed following the administration of laxatives
E. is effectively excluded by 3 negative stool samples

57. Women with systemic lupus erythematosus (SLE):

A.   are at no increased risk of miscarriage
B.   usually give birth to children with at least one abnormality
C.   have a recognised association when delivered of neonates with congenital heart block
D.   may take chloroquine safely in pregnancy
E.   have active disease if their ESR is elevated in pregnancy

58. Parkinson's disease:

A.   is associated with an increase in prevalence of dementia when compared with the general population
B.   produces frontal lobe cognitive defects
C.   produces significant clinical depression in 50% of patients with the condition
D.   patients with depression are more likely to have postural changes
E.   is associated with motor disability that does not correlate with mood abnormalities

59. The following statements about hyperaldosteronism are correct:

A.   the commonest cause of primary hyperaldosteronism is bilateral adrenal hyperplasia
B.   hypertension associated with hypokalaemia and reduced urinary potassium excretion is characteristic of hyperaldosteronism
C.   a rise in aldosterone in response to posture is more in keeping with adrenal hyperplasia than an adrenal adenoma
D.   adrenal venous sampling is required in all cases of primary hyperaldosteronism due to adrenal adenomas prior to surgery
E.   glucocorticoid-suppressible hyperaldosteronism is an autosomal dominant disorder

60. **The combined oestrogen and progestogen oral contraceptive:**

A.   has a protective effect against all ovarian cancers
B.   increases the risk of hepatocellular cancer
C.   increases the risk of endometrial cancer
D.   increases the risk of thromboembolic events dependent on the duration of use
E.   increases the risk of myocardial infarction in ex-users

Answers

1. A – F; B – F; C – F; D – T; E – F

TB is a notifiable disease, though there is significant under-reporting. Three negative smears are required to be considered not infectious. It is recommended that patients be isolated for the first two weeks of treatment only; AAFB are often visible in the sputum after this, but they are not viable. The algorithm for screening is complicated but some idea of the principles is advised [1]. Only about 5% of patients with AIDS in England and Wales develop TB [2].

1. British Thoracic Society. Control and prevention of tuberculosis in Britain: an updated code of practice. Br Med J. 1990;300:995–9.
2. Watson JM. Tuberculosis in Britain today. Br Med J. 1993;306:221–2.

2. A – F; B – T; C – F; D – T; E – F

Dermatomyositis (DM) and polymyositis (PM) are the most commonly acquired myopathies (excluding toxins) in developing countries. Diagnosis requires a compatible clinical picture, raised creatinine kinase activity, EMG changes and muscle biopsy showing necrosis and inflammation. DM produces a more acute onset of symptoms and is characterised by capillary damage on muscle biopsy. PM has a more insidious onset with no capillary damage. Arthralgia is common in DM, but rare in PM, only usually seen when there is associated interstitial lung disease.

Urbano-Marquez A, Casademont J, Gray JM. Polymyositis/dermatomyositis: the current position. Ann Rheum Dis. 1991;50:191–5.

3. A – T; B – T; C – F; D – T; E – F

Generalised tonic–clonic, absence, myoclonic, and atonic seizures are all examples of generalised epilepsy [1]. Rolling movements, gaze aversion, pelvic thrusting and asynchronous limb movements are all more typical of pseudoseizures as opposed to true epilepsy [2]. In the elderly, cerebrovascular disease is the commonest cause of recent-onset epilepsy [3]. Vigabatrin inhibits GABA transaminase whilst lamotrigine suppresses the release of glutamine [4].

1. Gram L. Epileptic seizures and syndromes. Lancet. 1990;336:161–3.
2. Howell SJL et al. Pseudostatus epilepticus. Q J Med. 1989;71:507–19.
3. Tallis R. Epilepsy in old age. Lancet. 1990;336:295–6.
4. Brodie MJ. Lamotrigine. Lancet. 1992;339:1397–400.

4.   A – T; B – T; C – T; D – F; E – T

SIAD is associated with a number of pulmonary and cerebral disorders (including acute psychosis), malignancy and drugs [1]. In many forms of SIAD, thirst is increased inappropriately. The characteristic findings are a high urinary osmolality relative to plasma osmolality, with increased urinary sodium excretion. Rapid administration of hypertonic saline may precipitate central pontine myelinolysis which may result in quadraparesis, bulbar palsy, coma and death.

1. Kovacs L, Robertson GL. Disorders of water balance – hyponatraemia and hypernatraemia. Ballière's Clin Endocrinol Metab. 1992;6(1):107–27.

5.   A – F; B – T; C – T; D – F; E – T

At least 20% of patients infected with hepatitis C develop cirrhosis [1]. Chronic infection is associated with cryoglobulinaemia, polyarteritis nodosa, a sicca-like syndrome, and membranoproliferative glomerulonephritis [2]. The risk of sexual transmission is low when compared with hepatitis B and HIV. Alpha interferon has been shown to improve serum transaminases, but relapse is common after treatment is discontinued.

1. Lau JYN, Davis GL. Managing chronic hepatitis C virus infection. Br Med J. 1993;306:469–70.
2. Johnson RJ et al. Membranoproliferative glomerulonephritis associated with hepatitis C virus infection. N Engl J Med. 1993;328:465–70.

6.   A – T; B – T; C – F; D – T; E – F

There are many causes of hair loss including infection, drugs, systemic illness and trauma [1]. Postpartum hair loss usually resolves within 18 months. In eunuchs, baldness does not occur unless they are receiving testosterone. Poor prognostic indicators in alopecia areata include onset in childhood, hair loss at the margins, nail involvement and an atopic state.

1.   Parkinson RW. Hair loss in women: what to say and do to ease these patients distress. Postgrad Med. 1992;91:417–22, 431.

7.   A – T; B – F; C – T; D – T; E – F

The 'a' wave is due to atrial systole. It is therefore prominent in TS, and in conditions that increase the right ventricular end diastolic filling pressure (RVEDP), such as ASDs. Obviously it is absent in AF. Cannon 'a' waves are seen in CHB where the RA contracts against a closed tricuspid valve. E is complete nonsense because the AV is on the left side of the heart.

Swanton RH. Cardiology. Blackwell Scientific Publications, London. 1989:9–10.

8.   A – T; B – T; C – F; D – F; E – T

Total cholesterol, triglycerides, LDL and VLDL cholesterol are typically raised in the nephrotic syndrome whilst HDL is reduced [1]. These changes occur because of an increase in hepatic cholesterol and lipoprotein synthesis, a reduction in peripheral and hepatic catabolism of serum lipoproteins, and an increase in urinary excretion of HDL. Diabetic nephropathy is the commonest cause of nephrotic syndrome and end-stage renal failure in the United States. Protein loading has been shown to increase urinary protein exchange and worsen hypoalbuminaemia [2]. Hypercoagulability is a recognised complication of the nephrotic syndrome.

1.   Carome MA, Moore Jr J. Nephrotic syndrome in adults: a diagnostic and management challenge. Postgrad Med. 1992;92:209–15, 218, 220.
2.   Kaysen GA. Albumin metabolism in the nephrotic syndrome: the effect of dietary protein intake. Am J Kidney Dis. 1988;12:461–80.

9. A – T; B – F; C – T; D – F; E – F

All sulphonylureas are metabolised in the liver [1,2]. Chlorpropamide
has the longest half-life of all sulphonylureas. It has been shown that
2.5 mg of glibenclamide given 30 minutes before breakfast is more
effective than 7.5 mg with breakfast [3]. Chlorpropamide and
glibenclamide have been incriminated in causing death due to
hypoglycaemia, particularly in the elderly and those with renal
impairment [4]. β-Blockers are relatively contraindicated in patients on
sulphonylurea or insulin therapy.

1. Ferner RE, Alberti KGMM. Sulphonylureas in the treatment of
    non-insulin-dependent diabetes. Q J Med. 1989;73:987–95.
2. Melander A et al. Sulphonylurea antidiabetic drugs. An update of their clinical
    pharmacology and rational therapeutic use. Drugs. 1989;37:58–72.
3. Sartor G et al. Improved effect of glibenclamide on administration before breakfast.
    Eur J Clin Pharm. 1982;21:403–8.
4. Ferner RE, Neil HAW. Sulphonylureas and hypoglycaemia. Br Med J.
    1988;296:949–50.

10. A – T; B – T; C – T; D – T; E – F

About 90% of symptomatic patients have a mild influenza-like illness
which is self-limiting [1]. Severe cases of Weil's disease may lead to
death from massive haemorrhage, renal or liver failure, or myocarditis.
The transient deterioration which is sometimes seen when penicillin is
given is known as the MacKay–Dick reaction [2]. Infected animals
usually remain well while excreting leptospira in their urine.

1. Ferguson IR. Leptospirosis update. Br Med J. 1991;302:128–9.
2. Ferguson I. Leptospirosis. Prescribers' J. 1991;31:185–9.

11. A – F; B – T; C – T; D – F; E – F

In GCA the kidneys, lungs and skin are rarely involved [1]. Blindness is
usually due to ischaemic optic neuritis but may be due to central retinal
artery occlusion, retrobulbar neuritis or cortical ischaemia [2]. The ESR
may not be elevated in up to about a quarter of patients [3]. Temporal
artery biopsy does not help in predicting outcome [4].

1. Hunder GG et al. The American College of Rheumatology 1990 criteria for the classification of giant cell arthritis. Arth Rheum. 1990;33:1122–8.
2. Reich KA et al. Neurologic manifestations of giant cell arteritis. Am J Med. 1990;89:67–72.
3. Paice EW. Giant cell arteritis: difficult decisions in diagnosis, investigation and treatment. Postgrad Med J. 1989;65:743–7.
4. Kyle V, Hazelman BL. Stopping steroids in polymyalgia rheumatica and giant cell arteritis. Br Med J. 1990;300:344–5.

12. A – F; B – F; C – T; D – F; E – F

LP is a treatment for benign intercranial hypertension, and is the way that the radiologist performs a myelogram in cord compression. LP is safe in SAH provided there is no focal neurology (although CT scans are the preferred investigation where such facilities exist, they are negative in 15% of SAH cases). Cerebellar signs are a common feature of MS, the diagnosis of which is aided by the finding of oligoclonal bands in the CSF.

Patten J. Neurological differential diagnosis. Harold Starke Ltd, London. 1977.

13. A – F; B – T; C – F; D – T; E – T

Growth hormone is secreted by acidophilic cells of the anterior pituitary gland. Its effects on growth occur via somatomedins which are produced in tissues and act locally. Somatomedin levels in malnutrition are low, but those of growth hormone are elevated. Nutritional status affects somatomedin action and thus the low somatomedin levels may influence growth hormone by negative feedback.

Zilva JF, Pannall PR, Mayne PD. Clinical chemistry in diagnosis and disease. Edward Arnold, London, 1988.

14. A – F; B – T; C – T; D – T; E – T

Factors predisposing to fractured NOF are related to bone strength – being female, oestrogen lack (i.e. B), and alcohol consumption predispose to osteoporosis. The risk of falling (i.e. D and E), and the neuromuscular response to falling are also important.

Anon. Fractured neck of femur: prevention and management. R Coll Phys, London. 1989.

15. A – T; B – F; C – T; D – T; E – F

An increasing number of inherited diseases can be diagnosed prenatally, allowing elective abortion. The same is true if there is maternal exposure to teratogens. There are no known acquired risks, which act via the father, that can be detected prenatally. The risks of abnormality become greater than the risk of intervention when the mother is aged over 35 years.

D'Alton ME, Decherney AH. Prenatal diagnosis. N Engl J Med. 1993;328(2):115–20.

16. A – F; B – T; C – F; D – T; E – T

There are 3 types of dissection in the DeBakey classification: type I involves the ascending and descending aorta; type II is confined to the ascending aorta; and type III is confined to the descending aorta [1]. Type III dissections are best treated medically initially. MRI scanning has been found to be a useful technique to evaluate a suspected aortic dissection but availability is a problem [2].

1. Treasure T, Raphael MJ. Investigation of suspected dissection of the thoracic aorta. Lancet. 1991;338:490–5.
2. Cigarroa JE et al. Diagnostic imaging in the evaluation of suspected aortic dissection. N Engl J Med. 1993;328:35–43.

17. A – F; B – F; C – T; D – T; E – T

The normal RBC lifespan is 120 days; this must be reduced for there to be a haemolytic anaemia. Because the bilirubin is unconjugated, it is not filtered by the glomeruli. In intravascular haemolysis the haemoglobin is bound by haptoglobin and the resulting complex is cleared by the reticulo-endothelial system in about 4 minutes. When this mechanism is saturated then haemoglobinuria occurs.

Tabbara IA. Haemolytic anaemias. Med Clin N Am. 1992;76(3):649–68.

18. A – F; B – F; C – T; D – T; E – F

Improvement in glycaemic control is the only therapeutic manoeuvre which has consistently been shown to retard the progression of diabetic neuropathy [1]. Full recovery from the amyotrophy usually occurs over a period of months. β-Blockers and diuretics tend to exacerbate impotence but not ACE inhibitors nor calcium channel blockers.

1. Dyck PJ. New understanding and treatment of diabetic neuropathy. N Engl J Med. 1992;326:1287–8.

19. A – F; B – F; C – T; D – F; E – T

Streptococcal pneumonia accounts for 60–75% of community-acquired pneumonias compared with *Mycoplasma pneumonia* (5–18%). There is a 21-fold increase in the risk of death or need for ITU when two or more of the following are present:

(i)   diastolic BP <60 mmHg
(ii)   respiratory rate >30/minute
(iii)   serum urea >7 mmol/L

Ciprofloxacin has poor activity against the pneumococcus, and erythromycin should be used as second line to tetracycline in psittacosis.

British Thoracic Society. Guidelines for the management of community-acquired pneumonia in adults admitted to hospital. Br J Hosp Med. 1993;49(5):346–50.

20. A – T; B – T; C – T; D – T; E – T

Intranasal calcitonin has been used in clinical trials but is not freely available as yet. Biphosphonates are potent inhibitors of bone resorption [1]. The dose of etridonate needed to inhibit bone resorption also impairs mineralisation of newly synthesised bone matrix. Other biphosphonates, such as pamidronate, inhibit resorption at concentrations which are much lower than that which impairs mineralisation. Side-effects of sodium fluoride include gastic irritation and a lower-extremity pain syndrome.

1. Riggs BL, Melton LJ. The prevention and treatment of osteoporosis. N Engl J Med. 1992;327:620–7.

21. A – F; B – T; C – F; D – F; E – T

The optic nerve is supplied by the ophthalmic artery which leaves the internal carotid directly, and divides into the choroidal and posterior ciliary branches. Occlusion of one of the subdivisions causes C which is typical. The main causes are arteritic, and non-arteritic; the main associations of the latter are DM and hypertension, so the patients tend to be >40. Slowly progressive disease implies compression of the optic nerve by a mass lesion.

Wray SH. The management of acute visual failure. J Neurol Neurosurg Psych. 1993;56:234–40.

22. A – F; B – T; C – T; D – F; E – F

Apart from the link with thyroid disease, the only known risk factor is smoking. Although not a predictor of severity of hyperthyroidism (it can occur in euthyroid patients), it tends to improve with treatment of hyperthyroidism. Since this is now detected earlier, the incidence seems to be falling.

Munro D. Thyroid eye disease. Br Med J. 1993;306:805–6.

23. A – F; B – F; C – T; D – T; E – F

Irritable bowel syndrome occurs more frequently in women than men. Those with diarrhoea predominantly have short colonic transit times, and those with constipation predominating have long transit times. Balloon distension of the rectum produces symptoms in 50–60% of patients compared with less than 10% of controls.

Zighelboim J, Talley NJ. What are functional bowel disorders? Gastroenterology. 1993;104:1196–1201.

24.   A – T; B – T; C – T; D – F; E – F

Specimens from mammoths have been analysed. A growing number of genetically determined diseases can be diagnosed with PCR (including muscular dystrophy). False-positive results can be obtained if similar sequences occur in unrelated nucleic acids. The main virtue of the technique is that, because it amplifies, only a small specimen is required; for this reason, it is not a good test for malaria when chronic low-grade parasitaemia is common in endemic areas.

Carman WF. The polymerase chain reaction. Q J Med. 1991;287:195–203.

25.   A – T; B – F; C – F; D – T; E – T

AF may be precipitated by acute hypovolaemia [1]. Lone AF is associated with a low risk of stroke [2]. β-Blockers are the drugs of choice in the treatment of AF secondary to thyrotoxicosis provided cardiac failure is not a problem [3]. Independent clinical predictors of an increased risk of stroke in subjects with non-rheumatic AF are:

(a)   recent (within 3 months) onset of CCF
(b)   history of hypertension
(c)   history of previous TIA or CVA

1. Edwards JD, Wilkins RG. Atrial fibrillation precipitated by acute hypovolaemia. Br Med J. 1987;294:283–4.
2. Pritchett ELC. Management of atrial fibrillation. N Engl J Med. 1992;326:1264–71.
3. Woeber KA. Thyrotoxicosis and the heart. N Engl J Med. 1992;326:94–8.
4. Hart RG. Cardiogenic embolism to the brain. Lancet. 1992;339:589–94.

26.   A – F; B – T; C – T; D – F; E – T

Serum erythropoietin is characteristically within or above the reference range, but is inappropriately low relative to the degree of anaemia in chronic renal failure [1]. Erythropoietin resistance occurs in the presence of decreased red cell production (as in iron deficiency or aluminium toxicity) or reduced red cell survival (as in blood loss or haemolysis) [2]. Indications for epoetin in patients with renal failure include angina or heart failure aggravated by anaemia, a previous requirement for regular blood transfusions, and withholding of transfusion to reduce sensitisation to transplantation antigens. Hypertension is often an early complication of PCKD and may precede the development of renal impairment [3]. Atenolol may accumulate in uraemic patients as it is cleared mainly by renal excretion.

1. Winearls C. Treatment of anaemia in renal failure. Prescribers' J. 1992;32:238–44.
2. Macdougall IC et al. Treating renal anaemia with recombinant human erythropoietin: practical guidelines and a clinical algorithm. Br Med J. 1990;300:655–9.
3. Raine AE. Management of hypertension in chronic renal failure. Prescribers' J. 1992;32:232–7.

27. A – T; B – T; C – F; D – F; E – F

Calcitonin has a rapid onset of action but its effect on serum calcium is not sustained with continued therapy [1]. Frusemide inhibits calcium reabsorption in the *ascending* limb of the loop of Henle. Emergency parathyroidectomy may be life-saving in acute severe hypercalcaemia if medical management is not improving the situation after 6–12 hours and there is no obvious cause for the hypercalcaemia from the initial clinical picture and investigations. Large parathyroid adenomas are often found under such circumstances.

1. Bilezikian JP. Management of acute hypercalcaemia. N Engl J Med. 1992;326:1196–203.

28. A – F; B – F; C – F; D – T; E – F

It is important to be clear about the various diseases that the four species of aspergillus can cause (allergic bronchopulmonary aspergillosis, aspergilloma and invasive aspergillosis being the most important). In invasive aspergillosis there is often no immune response (and therefore no serological test). It is not common in AIDS. Specialist advice should be sought on treatment but is usually a combination of amphotericin B, 5 flucytosine and itraconazole.

Wilson D, Denning DW. The commonest life-threatening mould infection: invasive aspergillosis. Hosp Update. 1993;19(4):225–33.

29. A – F; B – F; C – T; D – F; E – T

C is rheumatoid factor, which reacts against synovial cartilage, causing immune deposition. There is a HLA DR linkage with a consequent genetic association [1]. NSAIDs are not disease modifying agents, but can give considerable symptomatic relief. Hydroxychloroquine is one of several recognised disease modifying agents [2].

1. Sewell KL, Trentham DE. Pathogenesis of rheumatoid arthritis. Lancet. 1993;341:283–6.
2. Brooks PM. Clinical management of rheumatoid arthritis. Lancet. 1993;341:286–90.

30. A – F; B – T; C – T; D – F; E – T

Cluster headaches usually present in young men [1]. Pain may be accompanied by meiosis, ptosis, and oedema of the eyelid. Migraine tends to improve in the majority of women in the second and third trimesters [2]. Sumitriptan is a 5-HT$_1$ agonist which can be given either subcutaneously or orally [3].

1. Clough C. Non-migrainous headaches. Br Med J. 1989;299:70–2.
2. Lance JW. Treatment of migraine. Lancet. 1992;339:1207–9.
3. Bateman DN. Sumitriptan. Lancet. 1993;341:221–4.

31. A – F; B – F; C – T; D – F; E – T

IGT is diagnosed by the oral glucose tolerance test (WHO criteria) when the fasting venous plasma glucose is less than 7.8 mmol/L with a two hour post-75 g glucose load value of between 7.8 and 11.1 mmol/L [1]. (The figures for venous whole blood are 6.7, and 6.7–10.0 mmol/L respectively.) The annual risk of 'deterioration to diabetes' has been estimated to be between 2–10% [2]. Individuals with IGT have a doubling of risk of coronary heart disease and stroke. The risk of developing diabetic retinopathy in patients who remain in the IGT range is negligible. IGT is associated with hyperinsulinaemia and insulin resistance in both cross-sectional and longitudinal studies.

1. Keen H. The nature of the diabetic state. Med Int. 1989;65:2672–5.
2. Yudkin JS et al. Impaired glucose tolerance. Br Med J. 1990;301:397–402.

32. A – F; B – T; C – T; D – T; E – F

Advanced liver damage in PBC as assessed by histology may not correlate with the clinical and biochemical changes [1]. PBC may be associated with a number of other autoimmune disorders including Sjögren's syndrome, scleroderma, rheumatoid arthritis and fibrosing alveolitis. Ursodeoxycholic acid has been shown to improve both symptomatic and biochemical features of the disease [2]. PBC can recur after liver transplantation [3].

1. Mistry P, Seymour CA. Primary biliary cirrhosis – from Thomas Addison to the 1990s. Q J Med. 1992;299:185–96.
2. Bateson MC. New directions in primary biliary cirrhosis. Br Med J. 1990;301:1290–1.
3. Editorial. Is PBC cured by liver transplantation? Lancet. 1991;337:272–3.

33. A – F; B – T; C – T; D – T; E – F

Specific treatment is needed for aspirin ODs, but there is no antidote. The antidote for B, C and D are glucagon, Digibind Fab fragments, and i.v. calcium respectively.

Kulig K. Initial management of ingestions of toxic substances. N Engl J Med. 1992;326:1677–81.

34. A – T; B – F; C – T; D – T; E – F

Acute severe hypophosphataemia is recognised to occur in the treatment of diabetic ketoacidosis, chronic alcoholism and alcohol withdrawal, nutritional recovery, and recovery from hypothermia and severe burns [1]. There are diverse manifestations of severe hypophosphataemia including respiratory failure and encephalopathy. Oral phosphate therapy is generally preferred to intravenous because of the possibility of metastatic calcification [2].

1. Knochel JP. The pathophysiology and clinical characteristics of severe hypophosphataemia. Arch Intern Med. 1977;137:203–20.
2. Berkelhammer C, Bear RA. A clinical approach to common electrolyte problems: hypophosphataemia. Can Med Assoc J. 1984;130:17–23.

35. A – F; B – T; C – T; D – T; E – T

Dexfenfluramine is the dextrorotatory stereoisomer of fenfluramine, and has no stimulatory effects on the CNS in therapeutic doses as an appetite-suppressant [1]. Its main metabolite, d-norfenfluramine, is also active. Dexfenfluramine increases peripheral insulin sensitivity in both lean and obese subjects. Reversible pulmonary hypertension is a recognised adverse effect and the current advice is to prescribe the drug for no longer than 3 months at a time [2].

1. Finer N. Dexfenfluramine. Prescribers' J. 1993;33:16–21.
2. Committee on Safety of Medicines. Fenfluramine, dexfenfluramine and pulmonary hypertension. Curr Probl. 1992;34:1.

36. A – F; B – F; C – F; D – F; E – T

The main cells implicated in the inflammatory response are the eosinophil and the mast cell. Exacerbations are episodic and lung function usually returns to normal afterwards. Spirometry shows an obstructive defect, with reduced expiratory flow, with, traditionally, a 15% variability. Mortality is increasing. Frequent use of a β agonist is a marker of disease severity, and should be acted on.

McFadden ER, Gilbert IA. Asthma. N Engl J Med. 1992;327(27):1928–37.

37. A – T; B – T; C – T; D – F; E – F

The Guillain–Barré syndrome may present in a variety of ways. Demyelination as revealed on nerve conduction studies is said to be the most sensitive and specific laboratory finding in this condition. CSF protein is usually elevated, but if this is higher than 2.5 g/L then spinal cord compression becomes a more likely diagnosis. Corticosteroids have not been found to be useful in randomised controlled trials, but plasma exchange and intravenous immunoglobulin have [1,2].

1. Ropper AH. The Guillain–Barré syndrome. N Engl J Med. 1992;326:1130–6.
2. Guillain-Barré syndrome steroid trial group. Double-blind trial of intravenous methylprednisolone in Guillain-Barré syndrome. Lancet. 1993;341:586–90.

38. A – T; B – T; C – T; D – T; E – F

Drugs which have been implicated in the development of gynaecomastia include cimetidine, spironolactone, digoxin and cyproterone [1]. Oral testosterone has not been shown to be beneficial in the treatment of gynaecomastia, and indeed may worsen the condition through aromatisation to oestradiol.

1. Braunstein GD. Gynecomastia. N Engl J Med. 1993;328:490–5.

39. A – T; B – F; C – T; D – T; E – T

Acyclovir is a selective inhibitor of HSV types 1 and 2 and HVZ viruses [1]. It is ineffective in the treatment of CMV infections. It crosses the placenta and is concentrated in amniotic fluid. There have been no reports of fetal toxicity but the drug has only been used in a limited number of pregnancies. Acyclovir prophylaxis of HSV infections is beneficial in the severely immunocompromised, especially those undergoing bone marrow transplantations [2,3] or induction chemotherapy.

1. Whitley RJ, Gnann Jr JW. Acyclovir: a decade later. N Engl J Med. 1992;327:782–9.
2. Wade JC et al. Oral acyclovir for prevention of herpes simplex virus reactivation after marrow transplantation. Ann Intern Med. 1984;100:823–8.
3. Shepp DH et al. Sequential intravenous and twice-daily oral acyclovir for extended prophylaxis of herpes simplex virus infection in marrow transplant patients. Transplantation. 1987;43:654–8.

40. A – T; B – F; C – F; D – T; E – T

The heart's conduction system changes with age. Fifty percent of the sinus node in the young adult comprises pacemaker cells, which reduces to less than 10% after the age of 75. More than half of the left bundle branch may be replaced by fibrous tissue from the sixth decade. No specific age-related changes have been identified in the AV node or His bundle. In a series of 89 patients of 80 years or older, 50% of them had an improvement in dizziness or congestive cardiac failure. Pacemakers are sometimes required as a back-up when anticoagulants or anti-tachycardia drugs are needed by the patient.

MCQs for MRCP Part 1

Katritsis D, Camm AJ. Pacing in the elderly: where we stand now. Care of the elderly.
1991;3(8):379–82.

41. A – T; B – F; C – F; D – T; E – F

Primary PCV requires increased red cell mass, normal Pa O_2, and
either splenomegaly or two of thrombocytosis, leucocytosis, raised LAP
score or raised vitamin B_{12}. These secondary criteria are of course
indicative of a more generalised myeloproliferative process.

Berk PD et al. Therapeutic recommendations in polycythaemia vera based on
polycythaemia study group protocols. Semin Haematol. 1986;23:132–43.

42. A – T; B – F; C – T; D – F; E – F

Hyperglycaemia causes a shift of fluid from the intracellular to the
extracellular space, thus producing hyponatraemia. Up to 30% of
patients with ketoacidosis may have an initial serum potassium of
greater than 6 mmol/L [1]. Serum phosphate may drop to less than 0.32
mmol/L (which is considered to be potentially life-threatening) during
the treatment for ketoacidosis, but it has not been shown that giving
phosphate infusions 'prophylactically' improves morbidity or mortality
[2]. Bicarbonate therapy should only be considered if arterial pH is less
than 7.0, although some regard 6.9 as the 'action level' [3]. Leucocytosis
is common in ketoacidosis and may occur in the absence of infection.

1. Editorial. Hyperkalaemia in diabetic ketoacidosis. Lancet. 1986;2:845–6.
2. Keller U, Berger W. Prevention of hypophosphataemia by phosphate infusion during
   treatment of diabetic ketoacidosis and hyperosmolar coma. Diabetes. 1980;29:87–95.
3. Walker M et al. Clinical aspects of diabetic ketoacidosis. Diabetes Metab Rev.
   1989;5(8):651–63.

43. A – F; B – F; C – F; D – F; E – T

Although rare in this country it is a notifiable disease. The mode of
transmission is unknown and there is no known animal reservoir,
although it can be cultured in the footpad of the mouse and,
memorably, the armadillo. Working in a leprosy hospital gives 2–3 times
increased risk of contracting leprosy. It is the tuberculoid form which is

74

associated with an immune response.

Bryceson A. Leprosy. Medicine Int. 1992;107:4519–22.

44. A – T; B – F; C – F; D – F; E – F

The transmissible spongiform encephalopathies show similar pathological features in humans and animals. Part of the infectious agent is a prion protein which is a modification of a constituent of the normal cell membrane. Creutzfeldt–Jakob disease produces a rapid dementia, myoclonus and akinetic mutism, whereas Kuru produces progressive cerebellar ataxia followed by dementia later in the illness.

Esmonde TFG, Will RG. Transmissible spongiform encephalopathies and human neurodegenerative disease. Br J Hosp Med. 1993;49(6):400–6.

45. A – F; B – F; C – T; D – T; E – F

The polycystic ovarian syndrome (PCOS) is a common cause of hirsutism [1]. FSH:LH ratio is characteristically reduced in this condition [2]. Treatment of PCOS will depend upon the presentation: obese women will be helped by weight reduction; hirsutism may be managed by local physical treatments and hormonal manipulation (ethinylestradiol and cyproterone); infertility may be treated with clomiphene, LHRH, tamoxifen, laparoscopic ovarian diathermy, or wedge resection depending on the severity of the condition and response to previous therapy.

1.   Conway GS, Jacobs HS. Hirsutism. Br Med J. 1990;301:619–20.
2.   Barnes R, Rosenfield RL. The polycystic ovarian syndrome: pathogenesis and treatment. Ann Intern Med. 1989;110:386–99.

46. A – F; B – F; C – T; D – T; E – F

Few facts are always true in medicine but UC does always involve the rectum. Peak age is 20–40. Fibrosing alveolitis is a recognised association of both UC and sulphasalazine therapy. Sulphasalazine causes reversible oligospermia and should be avoided in men wishing to start a family, but is reckoned to be safe in pregnancy and childbirth.

Mills PR. Management of ulcerative colitis. Prescribers' J. 1993;33(1):1–7.

47. A – T; B – F; C – T; D – T; E – F

Renal impairment is present in 15–20% of patients who present with myeloma. It often improves with high fluid intake [1]. The single most important prognostic factor is the serum level of β_2-microglobulin at diagnosis [2]. There is some evidence to suggest that combination chemotherapy has advantages over intermittent melphalan with respect to long-term survival.

1. Winfield DA. Multiple myeloma. Br J Hosp Med. 1992;47:30, 32–4, 36–7.
2. Durie BGM et al. Prognostic value of pretreatment serum β_2-microglobulin in myeloma: a Southwest Oncology Group Study. Blood. 1990;75:823–30.
3. MacLennan ICM et al. Combined chemotherapy with ABCM versus melphalan for treatment of myelomatosis. Lancet. 1992;339:200–5.

48. A – F; B – T; C – F; D – F; E – F

Histology showing organising buds of connective tissue within the alveolar ducts is required to make the diagnosis, though BAL is recommended to exclude infection. Although steroids are generally effective, a negative response does not exclude the diagnosis.

Geddes DM. BOOP and COP. Thorax. 1991;46:545–7.

49. A – F; B – T; C – T; D – F; E – T

Oral gold and hydroxychloroquine have been found to be less effective than penicillamine, intramuscular gold, methotrexate and sulphasalazine in a meta-analysis of randomised controlled trials [1]. Thrombocytopenia associated with penicillamine therapy is a dose-related phenomenon. The risk of methotrexate hepatotoxicity is increased by antifolate drugs (such as cotrimoxazole), folic acid deficiency and renal impairment [2].

1. Felson DT et al. The comparative efficacy and toxicity of second-line drugs in rheumatoid arthritis. Arthritis Rheum. 1990;33:1449–61.
2. Brooks PM. Clinical management of rheumatoid arthritis. Lancet. 1993;341:286–90.

50. A – F; B – T; C – T; D – T; E – T

There is a sympathetically mediated rise in BP, heart rate and CO. Medullary compression causes parasympathetically mediated bradycardia. Myocardial ischaemia, thought to be catecholamine mediated, can occur as can ECG changes. Neurogenic pulmonary oedema is well known. There is an increase in metabolic rate causing increasing O_2 consumption.

Kaufman HH et al. Medical complications of head injury. Med Clin N Am. 1993;77(1):43–60.

51. A – T; B – T; C – F; D – F; E – F

Patients with solitary toxic nodules or toxic multinodular goitre are rarely kept in remission by antithyroid drugs [1]. There is no evidence for increased incidence of leukaemia following radioiodine. There is conflicting evidence as to whether radioiodine exacerbates thyroid eye disease or not. Carbimazole should be withdrawn 3–5 days before giving radioiodine so that uptake into the thyroid gland occurs. There may be a temporary exacerbation of thyrotoxic symptoms associated with the use of radioiodine because of further release of thyroid hormone, but this can be overcome by reinstituting carbimazole three days after the dose has been taken.

1. Franklyn J, Sheppard M. Radioiodine for hyperthyroidism. Br Med J. 1992;305:727–8.

52. A – F; B – T; C – F; D – T; E – F

Heterozygotes have no risks. Biliary copper excretion is reduced with copper retention and increased urinary excretion which leads to RTA (may be proximal or distal). In contrast to other chronic liver disorders, hepatoma is unusual.

Yarze JC et al. Wilson's disease: current status. Am Med J. 1992;92:643–54.

53. A – T; B – F; C – T; D – F; E – F

Reduced atmospheric pO_2 causes hyperventilation which leads to a compensatory HCO_3 excretion. Cardiac output is increased by increased rate for about a week. Rapid ascent is a risk factor for pulmonary and cerebral oedema. Retinopathy (usually haemorrhagic) requires ascent to very high altitude (>4500 m). Women are not advised to ascend to >2450 m in the first trimester.

Bezruchka S. High altitude medicine. Med Clin N Am. 1992;76(6):1481–97.

54. A – F; B – T; C – T; D – F; E – F

Echocardiograpic features of HOCM are: the ratio of the septal to posterior left ventricle wall of at least 1:3; the M-mode features of the left ventricle outflow tract; the systolic anterior motion of the mitral valve; and the premature systolic closure of the aortic valve.
The most important predictor of sudden death is the prescence of non-sustained ventricular tachycardia on holter monitoring. Amiodarone improves survival; class 1 antiarrhythmics and β-blockers do not prevent sudden death.

Odemuyiwa O, McKenna WJ. Problems in diagnosis and management of hypertrophic cardiomyopathy. Postgrad Med J. 1991;67:713–8.

55. A – F; B – T; C – T; D – F; E – T

It is exceptional for nephropathy to develop within 10 years of IDDM. Predictors are microalbuminuria, hyperfiltration, and rising blood pressure. Diabetics in ESRF have an increased mortality because of coronary and cerebral vascular disease. Progression can be slowed but not stopped by treatment of BP.

Breyer JA. Diabetic nephropathy in insulin-dependent patients. Am J Kidney Dis. 1992;XX(6):533–45.

56. A – T; B – T; C – F; D – F; E – T

Giardiasis is a common cause of the 'gay bowel syndrome' and can prove troublesome in patients with AIDS. Foul smelling flatulence is characteristic both in acute disease and afterwards; evidence of malabsorbtion can be found in 50% of *Giardia* patients. 76%, 90% and 97.6% of cases are found after 1, 2 and 3 stool samples respectively.

Wittner M, Tanowitz HB. Intestinal parasites in returned travellers. Med Clin N Am. 1992;76(6):1433–48.

57. A – F; B – F; C – T; D – F; E – F

There is a 40% increased risk of abortion via the cardiolipin syndrome. Most (i.e. >50%) children born to SLE mothers are normal but placental transmission of maternal antibodies can cause the 'transient neonatal lupus syndrome', with haematological and cardiac abnormalities ('C' = 38%). Chloroquine causes choroidoretinitis. The ESR rises in pregnancy anyway, and disease activity is preferably measured by C_3 activity.

De Swiet M. SLE and pregnancy. In: Seymour CA (ed). Horizons in Medicine No. 3. Royal College of Physicians, London. 1991:152–65.

58. A – T; B – T; C – F; D – T; E – T

70% of patients with Parkinson's disease suffer from at least one depressive symptom. However, only 10–25% actually have depression that fulfils vigorous diagnostic criteria. Mood abnormalities do not affect the degree of motor disability, but depression is seen more often in patients with gait and postural changes.

Ring H. Psychological and social problems of Parkinson's disease. Br J Hosp Med. 1993;49(2):111–6.

59. A – F; B – F; C – T; D – F; E – T

Seventy percent of cases of primary hyperaldosteronism are caused by an adrenal adenoma. There is inappropriately high urinary potassium excretion in the presence of hypokalaemia. Adrenal venous sampling is only indicated in difficult cases when other tests do not point to a single diagnosis [1]. In glucose-suppressible hyperaldosteronism [2], a paradoxical decrease in plasma aldosterone occurs in the postural study.

1. Case Records of the Massachusetts General Hospital. N Engl J Med. 1992;326:1617–23.
2. Editorial. Glucose-suppressible hyperaldosteronism. Lancet. 1992;339:1024–5.

60. A – F; B – T; C – F; D – F; E – F

The combined oral contraceptive has a protective effect against epithelial ovarian cancers, but not non-epithelial ovarian cancers. It increases the risk of hepatocellular cancer and adenoma, but reduces the relative risk of endometrial cancer. Myocardial infarction, thromboembolic events and subarachnoid haemorrhage all have an increased risk with use of the combined pill, but they are not affected by the duration of use and do not persist in ex-users.

Milne R, Vessey M. The pill and mortality – an overview. J Public Health Med. 1992;14(1):9–16.

Section 3 – Paediatrics

1. The preterm infant is at risk of:

A. persistent ductus arteriosus
B. necrotising enterocolitis
C. meconium aspiration
D. periventricular haemorrhage
E. polycythaemia

2. Recognised causes of acute stridor in children include:

A. hypocalcaemia
B. infectious mononucleosis
C. laryngomalacia
D. laryngotracheobronchitis
E. C1 esterase inhibitor deficiency

3. The following are features of neurofibromatosis type 1 in childhood:

A. axillary freckling
B. Lisch nodules
C. cardiac rhabdomyoma
D. shagreen patch
E. sphenoid dysplasia

4. Which of the following statements related to the molecular basis of cystic fibrosis are true:

A. F508 is the most frequent genotypic mutation in North European patients
B. the gene product is an exocrine cell membrane receptor
C. pancreatic insufficiency is not related to the genotype
D. ion transport regulation is defective
E. mutation analysis may be accomplished by using the polymerase chain reaction

5. **In the oral rehydration of infants with acute gastroenteritis:**

A. the rate of water absorption is influenced by the osmolality of the oral rehydration solution
B. inclusion of bicarbonate is essential for the correction of metabolic acidosis
C. amino acids aid electrolyte absorption
D. oral rehydration solutions contain sodium supplements at a concentration of 110 mmol/L
E. sucrose is superior to glucose

6. **Nephrotic syndrome in childhood:**

A. is usually due to membranous glomerulopathy
B. is characterised by generalized proteinuria
C. may be complicated by hypertension
D. may be the first manifestation of systemic lupus erythematosus
E. may be complicated by spontaneous bacterial peritonitis

7. **The following are features of Noonan's syndrome:**

A. coagulation defects
B. neck webbing
C. supravalvular aortic stenosis
D. X-linked inheritance
E. rockerbottom feet

8. **Radiological features particularly suggestive of non-accidental injury include:**

A. posterior rib fractures
B. metaphyseal fractures
C. clavicular fractures
D. parietal skull fractures
E. marked periosteal reaction

9. **The following are caused by human parvovirus B19 infection:**

A. roseola infantum
B. erythema infectiosum
C. hydrops fetalis
D. conjunctivitis
E. bone marrow aplasia in chronic haemolytic anaemia

10. **Classical congenital adrenal hyperplasia:**

A. is caused by 21-hydroxylase deficiency in over 90% of cases
B. is associated with salt-losing status in one-third of patients
C. is associated with an elevated 17-hydroxyprogesterone level
D. may be diagnosed antenatally
E. causes female infertility in treated cases

11. **Maternal polyhydramnios is associated with the following neonatal disorders:**

A. cystic adenomatoid malformation of the lung
B. myotonic dystrophy
C. Potter's syndrome
D. tracheoesophageal fistula with oesophageal atresia
E. congenital chloridorrhoea

12. **Which of the following are causes of prolonged neonatal conjugated hyperbilirubinaemia:**

A. congenital hypothyroidism
B. septo-optic dysplasia
C. Crigler–Najjar syndrome
D. extrahepatic biliary atresia
E. α_1-antitrypsin phenotype ZZ

13. Features of Kawasaki's disease include:

A. acute non-calculus hydrops of the gallbladder
B. thrombocytopenia
C. desquamation of fingers and toes
D. purpura
E. splenomegaly

14. Large-for-gestational-age infants are associated with:

A. gastroschisis
B. cardiomyopathy
C. hyaline membrane disease
D. polycythaemia
E. intra-abdominal malignancy

15. Recognised causes of childhood tall stature include:

A. homocystinuria
B. Soto's syndrome
C. Laron's syndrome
D. hypochondroplasia
E. neurofibromatosis type 1

16. Which disorders correlate with the accompanying classical electrolyte pattern?

A. hypokalaemic, hypochloraemic metabolic acidosis: pyloric stenosis
B. hyponatraemic, hypokalaemic metabolic acidosis: congenital adrenal hypoplasia
C. hyponatraemic, hypokalaemic metabolic alkalosis: Barrter's syndrome
D. metabolic acidosis with normal anion gap and urinary pH less than 5.5: primary proximal renal tubular acidosis
E. hypokalaemic, hypochloraemic metabolic alkalosis and elevated urinary chloride: congenital chloridorrhoea

17. Recognised causes of cyanotic heart disease include:

A. Ebstein's anomaly
B. tricuspid atresia
C. cor triatriatum
D. double outlet right ventricle with subpulmonary ventricular septal defect
E. hypoplastic left ventricle syndrome

18. The following are causes of neonatal vomiting:

A. congenital adrenal hyperplasia
B. necrotising enterocolitis
C. hypercalcaemia
D. congenital hypothyroidism
E. cow's milk protein intolerance

19. In paediatric HIV infection:

A. efficiency of vertical transmission is approximately 80%
B. persistence of HIV IgG antibody beyond 6 months of age is diagnostic
C. Kaposi's sarcoma is a rare malignancy
D. parotid enlargement often accompanies lymphoid interstitial pneumonitis
E. asymptomatic children can receive all standard immunisations

20. The following are more common in children with Down's syndrome:

A. congenital hypothyroidism
B. alopecia areata
C. cutis marmorata
D. imperfect canalisation of the nasolacrimal duct
E. coeliac disease

21. Chronic idiopathic thrombocytopenic purpura in childhood:

A. is defined as thrombocytopenia persisting beyond two months
B. occurs in 2–5% of of cases of acute ITP
C. usually necessitates splenectomy
D. may be treated with anti-D immunoglobulin
E. is a feature of systemic lupus erythematosus

22. Molluscum contagiosum:

A. is caused by a DNA virus of the poxviridae family
B. has an incubation period of two weeks to six months
C. requires no specific treatment
D. characteristically produces a vesicular rash with central umbilication
E. characteristically appears on extensor surfaces of the limbs

23. Which of the following statements concerning male phenotypic development are correct?

A. the Mullerian duct gives rise to the epididymis and vas deferens
B. the indifferent gonad is converted to a testis in response to a Y chromosome testis-determining gene
C. virilisation of the genital tubercle is under testosterone control
D. 5α-reductase deficiency causes the development of female external genitalia
E. urogenital sinus differentiates into the prostate and prostatic urethra

24. Chronic lung disease of prematurity (bronchopulmonary dysplasia):

A. may be diagnosed as oxygen dependence beyond two months of age
B. is due to surfactant deficiency
C. ventilator dependency may be reduced by the use of dexamethasone
D. may be complicated by ureaplasma infection
E. is associated with gastro-oesophageal reflux

25. In molecular biology:

A. Southern blot analysis detects protein composition
B. RNA splicing removes transcribed gene exons
C. RNA analysis is by Northern blot hybridisation
D. protein encoding areas of the gene are called introns
E. transcription occurs in a 3' to 5' direction along the gene

26. The *Haemophilus influenzae* type b (Hib) vaccination:

A. is a live attenuated vaccine
B. protects against non-encapsulated strains
C. may be given at the same time as the triple vaccine
D. is contraindicated in HIV-positive children
E. is given as a pre-school booster at the age of 5 years

27. A child of 18 months can:

A. build a tower of 6 cubes
B. turn pages in a book
C. cast objects
D. throw a ball without falling over
E. manage stairs two feet per step

28. Features of measles include:

A. incubation period of 14–21 days
B. petechiae visible on the soft palate
C. skin staining
D. Koplik's spots on the skin around the mouth
E. palmar desquamation

29. Ciprofloxacin:

A. is a monolactam antibiotic
B. is an oral anti-pseudomonal
C. has been associated with benign intracranial hypertension
D. is active against Chlamydiae
E. has no activity against Gram-positive organisms

30. The sweat test:

A. may be falsely positive due to the use of flucloxacillin
B. may be falsely positive in Cushing's syndrome
C. requires a total weight of sweat in excess of 100 mg
D. reveals a chloride concentration in excess of sodium concentration in cystic fibrosis
E. sum of sodium and chloride concentrations usually lies above 140 mmol/L in cystic fibrosis

31. Recognised causes of macrocephaly include:

A Canavan's disease
B. achondroplasia
C. neurofibromatosis type 1
D. Angelman's syndrome
E. congenital toxoplasmosis

32. Febrile convulsions:

A. occur in 10–15% of the childhood population
B. when recurrent occur in 33% of cases
C. have a positive family history in one-third of cases
D. occur up to the age of 10 years
E. are strongly correlated with the subsequent development of epilepsy

33. Congenital adrenal hypoplasia:

A. is associated with gonadotrophin deficiency
B. characteristically produces an elevated 17-hydroxyprogesterone level
C. has an X-linked inheritance
D. may be associated with an elevated creatine kinase
E. causes elevated urinary androgen levels

34. A normal six-month-old infant can:

A. transfer objects between hands
B. demonstrate a pincer grasp
C. sit unsupported
D. roll from prone to supine
E. feed himself with a spoon

35. Which of the following statements concerning meningococcal septicaemia are true?

A. septicaemia is usually accompanied by positive CSF cultures
B. blood cultures are positive in 80% of cases
C. septicaemia is mediated by endotoxins
D. it is usually accompanied by a maculopapular rash
E. hypotension is an early feature of septicaemic shock

36. Features of haemolytic–uraemic syndrome include:

A. prodromal diarrhoeal illness
B. burr cells on blood film examination
C. thrombocytosis
D. presence of Shigella verocytotoxins
E. peak incidence over 5 years

37. A white pupillary reflex is a feature of:

A. retinoblastoma
B. albinism
C. toxocariasis
D. retinopathy of prematurity
E. Aicardi's syndrome

38. Complications of phototherapy for neonatal hyperbilirubinaemia include:

A. cataracts
B. diarrhoea
C. macular rash
D. dehydration
E. bronze discolouration of skin

39. Ribavirin:

A. is a cytosine nucleoside analogue
B. is indicated in severe bronchiolitis due to respiratory syncytial virus
C. is teratogenic in humans
D. is administered as a small particle aerosol
E. has in vitro activity against influenzae and herpes viruses

40. Lyme disease in childhood:

A. is due to *Borrelia burgdorferi* spirochaete
B. IgM serology is available within the first week of infection
C. erythema marginatum occurs at the site of the tick bite
D. is treated with tetracycline therapy
E. aseptic meningitis occurs several weeks after infection

41. The following statements concerning the paediatric electrocardiograph are true?

A. a normal neonatal ECG has an electrical axis of $+60$ to $+180°$
B. T waves in V_2 lead are upright after 5 years of age
C. a short PR interval may be seen in glycogen storage disease II
D. left axis deviation occurs in pulmonary stenosis
E. PR elongation occurs with Ebstein's anomaly

42. Pauci-articular juvenile chronic arthritis:

A. is more common in females
B. occurs predominantly in late childhood
C. is erosive at small hand joints
D. is defined by the involvement of four or less joints
E. is associated with uveitis if antinuclear factor serology is negative

43. Neonatal periventricular leukomalacia:

A. is typically associated with grade III or IV intraventricular haemorrhage
B. is visible on cranial ultrasound within 10 days of birth
C. communicates with a horn of the lateral ventricle
D. may be associated with cerebral atrophy
E. carries a worse prognosis than a unilateral porencephalic cyst

44. **Recognised features of congenital hypothyroidism include:**

A. large posterior fontanelle
B. small for gestational age
C. inguinal hernia
D. dyshormonogenesis aetiology more common than glandular dysgenesis
E. prolonged unconjugated neonatal hyperbilirubinaemia

45. **Histopathological features of a jejunal biopsy in coeliac disease include:**

A. glandular hypoplasia
B. subtotal villous atrophy
C. lymphoid infiltration of the lamina propria
D. crypt hyperplasia
E. epithelioid granulomata

46. **Surfactant therapy for neonatal hyaline membrane disease is associated with:**

A. increased incidence of pulmonary haemorrhage
B. reduction in mortality in preterm infants
C. reduction in the incidence of periventricular haemorrhage
D. reduction in the incidence of pneumothorax
E. increased incidence of chronic lung disease (bronchopulmonary dysplasia)

47. **Typical features of marasmus are:**

A. advanced bone age
B. peripheral neuropathy
C. ascites
D. an increased mortality from measles
E. pellagra

48. **HIV-infected children should not receive the following vaccines:**

A. oral polio vaccine
B. measles mumps rubella vaccine
C. Hib vaccine
D. diphtheria vaccine
E. typhoid vaccine

49. **Roseola infantum:**

A. manifests as 'slapped cheek' syndrome
B. causes a high fever which settles as the rash appears
C. is caused by pleomorphic Gram-negative bacilli
D. is associated with peripheral desquamation
E. presents with conjunctivitis

50. **Features of sickle cell disease in children include:**

A. nocturnal enuresis
B. dactylitis
C. haemosiderotic cardiomyopathy
D. progressive splenomegaly
E. salmonella osteomyelitis

51. **Causes of intracranial calcification include:**

A. Rett's syndrome
B. kernicterus
C. congenital toxoplasmosis
D. tuberous sclerosis
E. craniopharyngioma

52. Maple syrup urine disease:

A. may present with seizures
B. presents with Gram-negative sepsis in one-third of cases
C. characteristically causes elevated urinary leucine, isoleucine and valine levels
D. is associated with hepatomegaly
E. may manifest as hypoglycaemia

53. Recognised features of Turner's syndrome include:

A. neonatal lymphoedema
B. hypoplastic nails
C. clinodactyly
D. increased incidence of antithyroid antibodies
E. horseshoe kidney

54. Necrotising enterocolitis:

A. only occurs in preterm infants
B. may be the presenting feature of Hirschsprung's disease
C. may appear radiologically as pneumatosis intestinalis
D. is associated with umbilical arterial catheter placement
E. may be associated with birth asphyxia

55. A serum calcium concentration of 3.2 mmol/L is compatible with:

A. Wilson's disease
B. William's syndrome
C. vitamin D intoxication
D. Di George syndrome
E. acute pancreatitis

56. **Deafness is a feature of:**

A. Pendred's syndrome
B. Waardenburg's syndrome
C. Turner's syndrome
D. Usher's syndrome
E. Hunter's syndrome

57. **Which of the following statements concerning infant nutrition are correct?**

A. decreased sodium content is a feature of preterm formula milk
B. hypocalcaemia is a feature of the early use of unmodified cow's milk
C. the use of cow's milk is associated with increased gastrointestinal blood loss
D. unmodified cow's milk has a high iron content
E. semi-skimmed cow's milk is advocated for children above 1 year

58. **Varicella infection:**

A. has an incubation period of 14–21 days
B. is a notifiable disease
C. may present initially with acute ataxia
D. remains infectious until there are no new crops of vesicles
E. is associated with marked thrombocytosis

59. **Constitutional delay in growth and puberty:**

A. is more common in females
B. is associated with dissonance of pubertal development
C. often features a positive family history
D. causes a disordered body segment pattern of long spine and short legs
E. is treated with recombinant growth hormone

60. A painful limp in a 3-year-old child may be due to:

A. slipped femoral epiphysis
B. neuroblastoma
C. Perthes' disease
D. irritable hip
E. Osgood–Schlatter disease

Answers

1. A – T; B – T; C – F; D – T; E – F

The preterm infant is born before 37 weeks' gestation. Preterm delivery is associated with multiple potential problems including: surfactant-deficiency hyaline membrane disease; neurological problems including periventricular haemorrhage; gastrointestinal disorders such as necrotising enterocolitis; hyperbilirubinaemia; anaemia; sepsis; metabolic disturbance (hypoglycaemia and hypocalcaemia) and patent ductus arteriosus. Meconium aspiration and polycythaemia are features of intrauterine growth retardation but not prematurity. The rare presence of meconium staining of the liquor in a preterm delivery strongly suggests perinatal sepsis, particularly listeriosis

2. A – T; B – T; C – F; D – T; E – T

Viral croup (laryngotracheobronchitis) is the most common cause of acute stridor in paediatrics. It is usually distinguishable from acute epiglottitis due to *Haemophilus influenzae* type b by the presence of a viral prodrome, barking cough and harsh stridor. Dysphagia, drooling and toxic appearance usually accompanies acute epiglottitis. Pharyngeal oedema due to infectious mononucleosis may cause acute stridor which is treated with steroid therapy. C1 esterase inhibitor deficiency causes recurrent acute stridor with angioedema. Inheritance is usually autosomal dominant. Fresh frozen plasma is required in the acute management. Laryngomalacia ('floppy larynx syndrome') causes chronic stridor.

Milner AD, Hull D (eds). Airways and lungs. In: Hospital paediatrics. Churchill Livingstone, Edinburgh. 1984.

3. A – T; B – T; C – F; D – F; E – T

Neurofibromatosis type 1, a gene defect mapped to chromosome 17, accounts for over 90% of neurofibromatosis cases in childhood.

97

Incidence is estimated at 1:3000–1:5000 and inheritance is autosomal dominant. Presentation of features is age dependent. Diagnostic criteria include: greater than six cafe au lait patches; two or more neurofibromata; axillary or inguinal freckling; optic glioma; two or more Lisch nodules (iris hamartomas); osseous dysplasia (e.g. pseudoarthrosis, sphenoid dysplasia) and an affected first-degree relative. Cardiac rhabdomyomas and shagreen patches are features of tuberous sclerosis.

Listerwick R, Charrow J. Neurofibromatosis type 1 in childhood. J Paediatr. 1990;116:845–51.

4.   A – T; B – F; C – F; D – T; E – T

The cystic fibrosis gene comprises 250 kilobases on chromosome 7q. The gene product, a polypeptide of 1480 amino acids, is termed the cystic fibrosis transmembrane regulator. The most common gene mutation (68% of Northern European patients) codes for a phenylalanine deletion at position 508. This may be detected using the polymerase chain reaction. Severe pancreatic insufficiency is correlated with the homozygous F508 genotype.

Tizzano EF, Buchwald M. Cystic fibrosis: beyond the gene to therapy. J Paediatr. 1992;120:337–49.

5.   A – T; B – F; C – F; D – F; E – F

The use of oral rehydration in gastroenteritis is a major advance in medicine. The important mechanism involves glucose-stimulated sodium transport into cells. Rehydration with improved renal perfusion usually corrects any metabolic acidosis without the need for bicarbonate supplements. There is no evidence for any beneficial effect from amino acids. In industrialised communities, the proprietary oral rehydration solutions contain a lower sodium concentration (approx-imately 60 mmol/L) to reduce the risk of accidental hypernatraemia.

Walker-Smith JA. Advances in the management of gastroenteritis in children. Br J Hosp Med. 1992;48(9):582–5.

6. A – F; B – T; C – T; D – T; E – T

Whilst nephrotic syndrome is often due to membranous glomerulopathy in adults, minimal change disease, associated with highly selective proteinuria, is much more common in children. SLE may present as nephrotic syndrome with membranous changes on renal biopsy. Complications include: hypovolaemia, which may present as hypertension due to intense vasoconstriction; infection due to relative immunosuppression; thrombosis; acute renal failure; hyperlipidaemia and malnutrition. Renal biopsy is not routinely performed. A third of steroid-responsive children never relapse, with a third having occasional steroid-responsive relapses and the rest remaining steroid dependent. The latter may need immunosuppressants or cytotoxic therapy.

Haycock GB. Nephrotic syndrome. Hospital Update. 1987;10:851–65.

7. A – T; B – T; C – F; D – F; E – F

Noonan's syndrome, inherited as an autosomal dominant, has an incidence of 1:1000–1:2000. There is a high spontaneous mutation rate. Typical facies include: hypertelorism, ptosis, depressed nasal bridge, low set ears and down-slanting palpebral fissures. Neck webbing occurs in 30%. 80–90% have cardiovascular defects – particularly right-sided lesions such as pulmonary stenosis. Skeletal defects occur in 95%. Coagulation defects of the intrinsic pathway occur in 54%. Supravalvular aortic disease occurs in William's syndrome. Rocker-bottom feet are seen in Edward's syndrome and Patau's syndrome.

Elsacri MM, Patton MA. Noonan syndrome. Mat Child Health. 1992;10:310–2.

8. A – T; B – T; C – F; D – F; E – T

No lesion is pathognomic of physical abuse. However, certain fractures are more likely to be due to such action. Metaphyseal injuries are often due to rapid acceleration/deceleration as in shaking. Rib fractures are usually occult and usually posterior resulting from thoracic compression. Periosteal bone formation results from subperiosteal haemorrhage. Birth trauma may cause clavicular fractures. Rarely metabolic bone

disease may cause confusion in the differential diagnosis of child
physical abuse. Linear narrow parietal skull fractures are findings of low
specificity for physical abuse. Fractures may be dated in relation to their
stage of healing which is of medicolegal importance.

Hobbs CJ. Fractures. In: Meadows R (ed). ABC of child abuse. Br Med J.
1989;298:1015–8.

9. A – F; B – T; C – T; D – F; E – T

The human parvovirus B19 is a DNA-containing virus. B19 associations
are: erythrocyte aplasia in chronic haemolytic anaemia; erythema
infectiosum (slapped-cheek syndrome; fifth disease); fetal infection
causing hydrops fetalis; arthropathy and vasculitic purpura. Erythema
infectiosum has an incubation period of 7–14 days and does not recur.
The sudden onset of red cheeks is accompanied by a generalised lacy
maculopapular rash. Diagnosis is serological by the demonstration of
anti-B19 IgM. Roseola infantum is caused by human herpes virus 6.

Ware R. Human parvovirus infection. J Paediatr. 1989;114:343–7.

10. A – T; B – F; C – T; D – T; E – F

Classical congenital adrenal hyperplasia is most commonly due to
21-hydroxylase deficiency. This enzyme defect, coded by two genes on
chromosome 6, prevents the conversion of 17-hydroxyprogesterone to
11-deoxycortisol, and progesterone to 11-deoxycorticosterone.
Two-thirds of cases are salt losers which, in the absence of sexual
ambiguity, may cause acute collapse. This is heralded by the initial rise
in serum potassium at the median of 4 days of age. Treatment is by
hormone replacement in the form of hydrocortisone and fludrocortisone
with salt supplementation. Sexual ambiguity requires a staged surgical
approach including clitoral reduction and vaginoplasty. Antenatal
diagnosis is possible with subsequent maternal dexamethasone
administration to reduce sexual ambiguity in female fetuses. Adequately
treated women are fertile although there is an increased incidence of
polycystic ovary syndrome.

Section 3 – Paediatrics – ANSWERS

Brook CGD. The management of classical congenital adrenal hyperplasia due to 21-hydroxylase deficiency. Clin Endocrinol. 1990;33:559–67.

11. A – T; B – T; C – F; D – T; E – T

Polyhydramnios is associated with gut obstruction; myotonic dystrophy; cystic adenomatoid lung malformation; neural tube defects; multiple pregnancy and congenital chloridorrhoea which is a secretory diarrhoea. Potter's syndrome of renal agenesis causes oligohydramnios. In any case of polyhydramnios, a nasogastric tube must be passed to exclude oesophageal atresia immediately after delivery.

12. A – F; B – T; C – F; D – T; E – T

Conjugated hyperbilirubinaemia is defined when 20% or more of the total bilirubin is conjugated. It is always pathological, indicating liver or biliary disease, and must be suspected in any infant in whom the urine is not colourless. The incidence is approximately 1:500 infants. Biliary atresia, with an incidence of 1:12 000, is a rare but important cause. Successful surgical treatment must be performed within 8 weeks of birth to prevent biliary cirrhosis, worsening portal hypertension and subsequent liver failure. α_1-Antitrypsin deficiency (phenotype ZZ) may be difficult to differentiate from biliary atresia. Septo-optic dysplasia includes mid-line defects, absent septum pellucidum and hypopituitarism. Hypothyroidism and Crigler–Najjar syndrome cause unconjugated hyperbilirubinaemia.

Mowat AP. Liver disorders in childhood. 2nd edn. Butterworths, London. 1987.

13. A – T; B – F; C – T; D – F; E – F

Kawasaki's disease has a peak incidence at 9–12 months of age; it is rare beyond 8 years. The aetiology is uncertain; there is a slight male preponderance and a distinct oriental prevalence. There is no diagnostic test. Diagnostic criteria include: fever for at least 5 days; bilateral conjunctival infection; polymorphous rash (often exacerbated in the perineum); cervical nodes; peripheral changes such as oedema or

101

desquamation and changes in the oral mucosa/tongue. Gallbladder
hydrops occurs in 3%. Thrombocytosis appears in week two and peaks
in the third week. Cardiovascular complications occur in up to 30%.
Coronary artery vasculitis may cause aneurysms which may persist.
Early therapy with gammaglobulin and aspirin reduces coronary artery
involvement.

Nadel S, Levin M. Kawasaki disease. In: David TJ (ed). Recent advances in paediatrics.
Churchill Livingstone, Edinburgh. 1993:103–16.

14. A – F; B – T; C – T; D – T; E – T

Large size for gestational age is often due to hyperinsulinism. Infants of
diabetic mothers have hyperinsulinaemia causing hypoglycaemia. As a
growth factor, insulin leads to polycythaemia with the subsequent risk of
jaundice and hyperviscosity syndrome. Insulin prevents surfactant
production so hyaline membrane disease is more common. A
cardiomyopathy, amenable to propranolol therapy, occurs in infants of
diabetic mothers. Exomphalos (not gastroschisis), large size and
predisposition to intra-abdominal malignancy are a feature of
Beckwith–Weidemann syndrome. Other features of
Beckwith–Weidemann syndrome are: macroglossia, abnormal ear
grooves, peripheral lymphoedema and pancreatic islet cell hyperplasia.

15. A – T; B – T; C – F; D – F; E – F

Familial tall stature is the most common cause. Homocystinuria is
phenotypically similar to Marfan's syndrome but, in addition, features
some mental retardation and a predisposition to vascular
thromboembolic episodes. Soto's syndrome comprises large babies who
continue to grow fast although subsequent growth deceleration prevents
excessive final height. Macrocrania, mild non-progressive
hydrocephalus, mental retardation and predisposition to various
malignancies are other features. Laron's syndrome (growth hormone
receptor abnormality) and hypochondroplasia are causes of short
stature. Short stature is an inconsistent feature of neurofibromatosis.

Westphal O. Tall stature. Growth Matters. 1991;8:2–4.

16. A – F; B – F; C – T; D – T; E – F

Pyloric stenosis may be complicated by a hypokalaemic, hypochloraemic metabolic alkalosis. Congenital adrenal hypoplasia may be present with an electrolyte pattern identical to that seen in congenital adrenal hyperplasia. Differentiation is aided by the absence of raised steroid precursors such as 17-hydroxyprogesterone. Due to high faecal chloride loss, urinary chloride levels are negligible in congenital chloridorrhoea.

17. A – T; B – T; C – F; D – T; E – T

The more common cyanotic lesions are: great vessel transposition, pulmonary atresia and Fallot's tetralogy. Ebstein's anomaly occurs in less than 1% of congenital heart disease and some cases are associated with maternal lithium use during early pregnancy. Whilst not classically cyanotic, hypoplastic left ventricle disease is associated with arteriovenous mixing and therefore the baby is slightly blue. The classical picture is of fulminant heart failure which may be mistaken for septicaemia. Cor triatriatum is a rare acyanotic lesion where a membrane divides the left atrium into two chambers and restricts flow from the pulmonary veins into the left ventricle.

Jordan SC, Scott O. Heart disease in paediatrics. 3rd Edn. Butterworths, London. 1989.

18. A – T; B – F; C – T; D – F; E – F

Salt-losing crisis in male infants with 21-hydroxylase-deficient congenital adrenal hyperplasia is an important cause of vomiting in the second and third week of life. Necrotising enterocolitis presents as abdominal distension, bloody stools, peritonitis, visceral perforation and apnoeic episodes. Congenital hypothyroidism causes increased gut transit time. Loose stools, sometimes bloody, are seen in cow's milk protein intolerance. Other important causes of vomiting include pyloric stenosis, gastrointestinal atresia/stenosis, sepsis and metabolic disease.

19. A – F; B – F; C – T; D – T; E – F

Most children acquire HIV infection through vertical transmission which has an efficiency of about 13%. Diagnosis in infants is difficult (unreliable IgM) but persistence of IgG beyond 18 months suggests infection and not transplacental passage of maternal IgG. Less than 4% of children develop Kaposi's sarcoma. Lymphoid interstitial pneumonitis may be associated with polyglandular enlargement unlike pneumocystis infection. Infants presenting with *Pneumocystis carinii* pneumonia have a worse prognosis than those with interstitial pneumonitis. BCG vaccination is contraindicated in HIV-infected children.

Mok JYQ. Management of HIV infection. In: David TJ (ed). Recent advances in paediatrics. Churchill Livingstone, Edinburgh. 1992:1–19.

20. A – T; B – T; C – T; D – T; E – T

Other conditions seen more frequently in Down's syndrome include: congenital heart disease; growth retardation; hypotonicity; hyperkeratotic skin; vitiligo; hypermetropia; deafness; duodenal atresia; leukaemia; epilepsy and early dementia.

Newton RW, Newton JA. Management of Down's syndrome. In: David TJ (ed). Recent advances in paediatrics. Churchill Livingstone, Edinburgh. 1992:21–35.

21. A – F; B – F; C – F; D – T; E – T

Chronic ITP arises in 10–20% of cases of acute ITP; it is defined as thrombocytopenia persisting beyond six months. Spontaneous recovery may still occur years later. Splenectomy will cure two-thirds of sufferers but at the increased risk of encapsulated organism septicaemia. It is rarely recommended for children. Temporary elevation of platelet count may be accomplished by steroids or intravenous gammaglobulin. Other therapies include: danazol, anti-Rhesus D immunoglobulin, vitamin C and cytotoxic drugs. The risk of intracranial haemorrhage is less than 1%.

Eden OB, Lilleyman JS. Guidelines for management of idiopathic thrombocytopenic purpura. Arch Dis Child. 1992;67:1056–8.

22. A – T; B – T; C – T; D – F; E – F

Infection usually resolves within a year. It is rare on palms, soles and mucous membranes. It is a papular rash with central umbilication. Contact sports, swimming pools and shared towels should be avoided.

Highet AS. Molluscum contagiosum. Arch Dis Child. 1992;67:1248–9.

23. A – F; B – T; C – F; D – T; E – T

Mullerian-inhibiting hormone causes Mullerian ducts to regress. The Wolffian duct gives rise to the vas deferens and epididymis. Testosterone is the principal androgen but dihydrotestosterone controls the virilisation of external genitalia and urogenital sinus. Dihydrotestosterone mediates most of the male pubertal changes termed secondary sexual features. 5α-reductase deficiency is an autosomal recessive disorder. The features are of dihydrotestosterone deficiency–female phenotype until virilisation at puberty.

Griffin JE. Androgen resistance – the clinical and molecular spectrum. N Engl J Med. 1992;326(9):611–18.

24. A – F; B – F; C – T; D – T; E – T

Chronic lung disease is defined as oxygen dependence beyond four weeks of age and has a multifactorial aetiology including: barotrauma, oxygen toxicity, pulmonary oedema and infection. 15–45% of infants under 1500 g ventilated for hyaline membrane disease develop chronic lung disease. Dexamethasone is of benefit in ventilator dependence. Diuretics improve lung mechanics; theophyllines augment diuretics and act as respiratory stimulants. Prevention is by reducing preterm delivery, length of ventilation and reduction in ventilator pressure.

Cameron D. Bronchopulmonary dysplasia. Hosp Update. 1992;11:814–21.

25. A – F; B – F; C – T; D – F; E – F

Southern blot analysis is used for restriction endonuclease cleaved DNA. Genes contain exons and introns. Transcription (5' end to 3' end) is followed by intron removal by RNA splicing. Exons contain protein coding information.

Latchman DS. Gene regulation. Br Med J. 1992;304:1103–5.

26. A – F; B – F; C – T; D – F; E – F

The Hib vaccine is a conjugate of capsular polysaccharides to various immunogenic proteins. It protects against invasive encapsulated strains responsible for acute epiglottitis and meningitis. Current recommendations suggest 3 doses of Hib vaccine; if over 13 months of age, just one dose of Hib vaccine is given. As the incidence of invasive disease decreases sharply after the age of 4, there is no need for a pre-school booster. As it is not a live vaccine, it is not contraindicated in HIV disease.

Immunisation against infectious disease. HMSO, London. 1992:44–9.

27. A – F; B – T; C – F; D – T; E – T

A child of this age can build a tower of 3–4 cubes. Casting of objects has ceased. Stairs can be negotiated and the child can seat himself in a chair. He will manage a spoon and can point to 3 parts of the body on request.

Illingworth RS. Basic developmental screening 0–4 years. 4th Edn. Blackwell Scientific Publications, Oxford. 1988.

28. A – F; B – F; C – T; D – F; E – F

Measles has an incubation period of 1–2 weeks. A prodromal period is followed by coryza, conjunctivitis, fever and Koplik's spots on the buccal mucosa. The maculopapular rash commences behind the ears then spreads, becoming confluent in 2 days. Diapedesis gives rise to some purpura followed by skin staining. Mild desquamation, sparing the palms, may follow. Upper respiratory involvement may be sufficient to cause croup. Palatal petechiae are more commonly seen in rubella or infectious mononucleosis.

29. A – F; B – T; C – T; D – T; E – F

Ciprofloxacin is a fluoroquinolone antibiotic. It has both Gram-positive and -negative spectra including *Pseudomonas* species. Some chlamydiae and rickettsiae are sensitive. Its use in children has been associated with several adverse reactions involving joints, kidneys and CNS. There is animal data to suggest toxicity to joint cartilage. It is related to nalidixic acid.

Archivist. Ciprofloxacin toxicity. Arch Dis Child. 1992;67:1285.

30. A – T; B – F; C – T; D – T; E – T

There are many causes of a false positive sweat test including: adrenal insufficiency, flucloxacillin therapy, ectodermal dysplasia, nephrogenic diabetes insipidus, hypothyroidism, glycogen storage disease type I and mucopolysaccharidoses. Normal subjects have sweat tests with sodium content above that of the chloride concentration.

David TJ. Cystic fibrosis. Arch Dis Child. 1990;65:152–7.

31. A – T; B – T; C – T; D – F; E – F

The most common cause of macrocephaly is familial. Other common causes of abnormally large head size are either hydrocephalus or subdural collections of fluid. Hydrocephalus may be caused by posterior fossa cerebral tumours. Progressive neurodegeneration associated with excessive accumulation of abnormal substances e.g. Tay–Sachs, Canavan's disease may cause megalencephaly (excessive brain mass). This may be associated with neurofibromatosis type 1. Platybasia with differential growth of skull bones results in the typical skull shape seen in achondroplasia. Angelman's syndrome, a microdeletion on

chromosome 15q, causes microcephaly, as does congenital
toxoplasmosis.

Weiner HL, Urion DK, Levitt LP. Paediatric neurology for the house officer. 3rd Edn.
Williams and Wilkins, Baltimore. 1988:23–32.

32. A – F; B – T; C – T; D – F; E – F

Febrile convulsions occur in 3% of the population between the ages of 6
months and 6 years. Recurrence occurs in one-third and is more likely
in those who develop seizures in early life. There is a positive family
history in up to one-third of cases. Seizures which are generalised
lasting less than 15–20 minutes are not associated with increased risk of
epilepsy. Risk increases with atypical prolonged seizures. Febrile
seizures may be the presenting feature of meningitis, in the absence of
other signs, in those under 18 months, so admission and lumbar
puncture must be seriously considered. Anticonvulsant prophylaxis is
rarely indicated, whilst home-rectal diazepam may be useful.

Joint working group of the research unit of the Royal College of Physicians and the
British Paediatric Association. Guidelines for the management of convulsions with fever.
Br Med J. 1991;303:634–6.

33. A – T; B – F; C – T; D – T; E – F

Congenital adrenal hypoplasia is a rare condition of X-linked, sporadic
or autosomal recessive inheritance. Presentation is usually acute
collapse of a male infant in a manner similar to that seen in congenital
adrenal hyperplasia. 17-Hydroxyprogesterone and urinary androgen
levels are low. Congenital adrenal hypoplasia has been associated with:
icthyosis, gonadotrophin deficiency, muscular dystrophy and deafness.

Sachmann M, Fuchs E, Prader A. Progressive high frequency hearing loss: an additional
feature in the syndrome of congenital adrenal hypoplasia and gonadotrophin deficiency.
Eur J Pediatr. 1992;151:167–9.

34. A – T; B – F; C – T; D – F; E – F

A 6-month-old infant sits unsupported although the arms may provide some propping. Rolling from supine to prone begins but not vice versa which begins at 7–8 months. Casting of objects and following their descent commences at one year. A pincer grasp is not seen until 9 months of age. A palmar grasp is evident at 6 months.

Illingworth RS. Basic developmental screening 0–4 years. 4th Edn. Blackwell Scientific Publications, Oxford. 1988.

35. A – F; B – F; C – T; D – F; E – F

Meningococcal septicaemia may occur without meningitis. Mortality approximates to 40%. The classical rash is petechiae/purpura although a proportion present as a maculopapular rash. Blood cultures are positive in less than 50% of cases; the organism may be grown from nasal swabs. Rapid antigen latex agglutination tests are positive in less than 70% of cases. Endotoxinaemia causes capillary leak, hypovolaemia and platelet activation. Hypotension appears late.

Heyderman RS, Klein N, Levin M. Pathophysiology and management of meningococcal septicaemia. In: David TJ (ed). Recent advances in paediatrics. Churchill Livingstone, Edinburgh. 1993:1–18.

36. A – T; B – T; C – F; D – F; E – F

Haemolytic–uraemic syndrome in childhood occurs predominantly between the ages of 3 months and 3 years. Many cases follow a viral-type diarrhoeal disease although some seem to be sporadic. The cause seems to be verocytotoxins produced by strains of *Escherichia coli*, particularly 01457:H7. Shigella may produce a similar but distinct illness. Haemolysis and thrombocytopenia occur due to microangiopathic thrombocytopenia/haemolytic anaemia. Usually there is uraemia and hyperbilirubinaemia without evidence of disseminated intravascular coagulopathy. Blood film reveals marked red cell fragmentation – 'burr' cells. The acute epidemic form, occurring in summer after a 'viral' diarrhoeal illness, has a better prognosis than the sporadic type.

Treatment is with plasma and renal support should acute renal failure intervene.

Milford DV, Taylor CM. New insights into the ℓaemolytic uraemic syndrome. Arch Dis Child. 1990;65:713–6.

37. A – T; B – F; C – T; D – T; E – F

A white pupillary reflex (leukocoria) is uncommon. Possible causes include: retinoblastoma, endophthalmitis, retinopathy or prematurity, cataract, toxocariasis and congenital abnormalities. Aicardi's syndrome comprises severe mental retardation, infantile spasms, agenesis of the corpus callosum and vertebral anomalies; chorioretinitis occurs and does not cause leukocoria.

38. A – F; B – T; C – T; D – T; E – T

Phototherapy is indicated for neonatal unconjugated hyperbilirubinaemia. Blue light (wavelength 400–500 nm) causes photoisomerization of bilirubin to a more water-soluble form which can then be excreted without conjugation. It is not recommended for conjugated hyperbilirubinaemia which may result in skin bronzing. Adverse effects include: fluid loss, maternal anxiety leading to reduced or difficult bonding, a photosensitive macular rash and diarrhoea due to increased faecal water loss plus changes in gut prostaglandin physiology. Phototherapy reduces skin bilirubin so the subsequent skin colour is not a good indicator of serum bilirubin.

Maisals MJ (ed). Neonatal jaundice. Clin Perinatol. WB Saunders, Philadelphia. 1990;17:2.

39. A – F; B – T; C – F; D – T; E – T

Ribavirin is a guanosine analogue. It is indicated for the treatment of respiratory syncytial virus bronchiolitis. It is given as a small particle aerosol. It has in vitro activity against several viruses and has been used, experimentally, in adenovirus, measles and viral haemorrhagic fever infections. No human teratogenicity has been noted but the drug can be detected in the urine of nursing staff up to weeks after occupational exposure. Its mode of action is probably interference with the guanylation step required for 5′ capping of the viral messenger RNA.

Barry W, Cockburn F, Cornall R et al. Ribavirin aerosol for acute bronchiolitis. Arch Dis Child. 1986;61:593–7.

40. A – T; B – F; C – F; D – F; E – T

Lyme disease, caused by the spirochaete *Borrelia burgdorferi*, is transmitted by tick bites – by the genus *Ixodes* in the UK. The classical spreading rash of erythema chronicum migrans occurs at the site of the tick bite. Blood serology is of little value in the first couple of weeks. Delayed diagnosis can lead to: aseptic meningitis, cranial polyneuropathy, myocarditis, arthritis and myositis. Early treatment with erythromycin and penicillin is effective. Tetracyclines are relatively contraindicated in children. Severe Lyme disease requires parenteral penicillin or third-generation cephalosporins.

Cryan B, Wright DJM. Lyme disease in paediatrics. Arch Dis Child. 1991;66:1359–63.

41. A – T; B – T; C – T; D – F; E – T

The usual ECG axis at birth is +135°. Left axis deviation is associated with tricuspid atresia, ventricular septal defect and endocardial cushion defects. The T wave inverts after 3 days in leads V4R and V1; the inverted T waves in leads V2 and V3 become upright after 5 years of age. PR interval elongation occurs with atrioventricular septal defect, Ebstein's anomaly, myotonic dystrophy and cardiomyopathy. Short PR intervals occur in Wolff–Parkinson–White, Lown–Ganong–Levine syndromes, Duchenne muscular dystrophy, Pompe's disease and hypertrophic obstructive cardiomyopathy.

42. A – T; B – F; C – F; D – T; E – F

Pauciarticular juvenile chronic arthritis occurs predominantly in young girls, with four or less joints affected. Affected joints are large, e.g. knees, and the disease is usually non-erosive. It is rheumatoid factor negative. Pauciarticular disease comprises 65% of childhood JCA. Fifty percent have positive antinuclear autoantibodies. Eighty percent of children with positive antinuclear autoantibodies have uveitis. Slit lamp screening is mandatory in such circumstances. Treatment is largely symptomatic using non-steroidal anti-inflammatory agents such as naproxen.

Craft AW. Arthritis in children. Br J Hosp Med. 1985;33:188–94.

43. A – F; B – F; C – F; D – T; E – T

Periventricular leukomalacia is a cystic degeneration of periventricular white matter developing after an ischaemic episode. Cysts are usually small (< 1 cm) and may coalesce. They do not usually communicate with a lateral ventricle unlike a porencephalic cyst which results from a venous infarct. Periventricular leukomalacia is not necessarily associated with severe intraventricular haemorrhage. Cerebral atrophy may accompany cyst formation. Neurodevelopmental problems are often marked particularly if bilateral or mainly occipital. The neurodevelopmental significance of porencephalic cysts is controversial although cerebral palsy may occur.

Levene MI. Cerebral ultrasound and neurological impairment: telling the future. Arch Dis Child. 1990;65:469–71.

44. A – T; B – F; C – F; D – F; E – T

Only 5% of cases of congenital hypothyroidism clinically manifest in the first week of life. Features include: large posterior fontanalle; dry skin; bradycardia; macroglossia; size greater than 4 kg; prolonged unconjugated hyperbilirubinaemia; umbilical hernia; hoarse cry; coarse facies and constipation. Neonatal screening measures TSH elevation so a pituitary cause may be missed. Glandular dysgenesis accounts for about 85% of cases with dyshormonogenesis 10%. The lower the original T4 level, the more severe is the case. These are usually cases of athyreosis. Bone maturation is usually delayed. Despite adequate T4 replacement, the TSH level may fail to return to 'normal' levels for several months. Incidence is 1:4000–1:6000 but is much more common in the Down's syndrome population (1:150–1:200).

45. A – F; B – T; C – F; D – T; E – F

The histopathological appearances of coeliac disease on jejunal biopsy are subtotal villous atrophy and crypt elongation/hyperplasia. Increased villous cell loss is accompanied by a compensatory increase in crypt cell replication. The columnar epithelial cells become pseudostratified or cuboidal. There is an increase in plasma cells in the lamina propria with a concomitant decrease in lymphocytes. Epithelioid granulomata occur in Crohn's disease.

Walker-Smith JA, Phillips AD. Small intestinal enteropathies. In: Milla PJ, Muller DPR (eds). Harries paediatric gastroenterology, 2nd Edn. Churchill Livingstone, Edinburgh. 1988:182–196.

46. A – T; B – T; C – F; D – T; E – F

Hyaline membrane disease is associated with surfactant deficiency. Exogenous surfactant replacements using both natural and artificial surfactants have been investigated recently. The majority of studies have identified a reduction in preterm infant mortality, particularly in smaller babies. The effects of surfactant in larger babies or those with alternative diagnoses remains in question. An increased incidence in pulmonary haemorrhage has been noted. This may be due to persistence of a patent ductus arteriosus with the production of blood-stained pulmonary oedema. The effect on pneumothoraces seems to be reduced whilst that of periventricular haemorrhage is debated but no evidence of reduction in incidence is yet apparent. The morbidity of chronic lung disease is as yet unchanged. Natural surfactant works faster than artificial, e.g. Exosurf; the latter may provide a substrate pool for surfactant production rather than having a direct effect.

Cooke R. Lung surfactant in newborns. Hosp Update. 1992;12:847–8.

47. A – F; B – F; C – F; D – T; E – F

Marasmus, nutritional deficiency due to poor intake of an essentially
normal balanced diet, differs clinically from kwashiorkor despite both
being encompassed by the term protein–energy malnutrition. Marasmic
features include low weight, fat and muscle wasting with increased
susceptibility to infection. Loss of appetite occurs with kwashiorkor
whereas it is rare in marasmus. Biochemical abnormalities are less than
with kwashiorkor. Ascites, oedema and low serum albumin are features
of kwashiorkor. Any such state leads to increased mortality from
measles but this has been reduced by vitamin A supplementation.
Pellagra, due to niacin deficiency, rarely accompanies marasmus.
Neuropathy is a feature of infantile beri beri – the acute form may
resemble kwashiorkor due to oedema resulting from cardiac failure.
Skeletal maturation and bone age estimation are delayed.

48. A – F; B – F; C – F; D – F; E – F

HIV-infected children should receive all standard immunisations with
the exception of BCG. There are reports of disseminated BCG infection
in such cases. However HIV status is not currently a prerequisite prior
to routine neonatal BCG vaccination. Whilst oral polio vaccine is not
strictly contraindicated in HIV-infected children, it is probably
preferable to use inactivated oral polio vaccine to minimise the risk of
polio infection in any immunocompromised family members.

Immunisations against infectious disease. HMSO. 1992:9.

49. A – F; B – T; C – F; D – F; E – F

Roseola infantum, one of the exanthemata, is caused by human herpes
virus type 6. Characteristically the high fever begins to subside when the
macular rash appears. It is not associated with peripheral desquamation
unlike group A streptococcal disease, Kawasaki's disease and, rarely,
measles. Initial leukocytosis may change to leukopenia and
lymphocytosis. Conjunctivitis is a feature of measles and some
adenovirus infections.

50. A – T; B – T; C – F; D – F; E – T

Sickle cell disease often presents as one of several forms of crisis: painful, infective, sequestrative, aplastic or chest syndrome. Painful crises may initially manifest in young children as 'hands and feet' syndrome – dactylitis. Sequestration, particularly splenic, occurs in infancy with acute splenomegaly. However recurrent splenic infarcts cause 'autosplenectomisation' with the absence of a palpable spleen in early childhood. Infective crises may be caused by unusual organisms. Osteomyelitis due to salmonellae is well recorded. Disease affecting the renal medulla, and consequently the concentrating power of the kidneys, gives rise to nocturnal enuresis. Haemosiderotic cardiomyopathy is a feature of haematological disorders requiring multiple transfusions and subsequent iron overload such as B thalassaemia.

Evans JPM. Practical management of sicke cell disease. Arch Dis Child. 1989;64:1748–51.

51. A – F; B – F; C – T; D – T; E – T

There are many causes of intracranial calcification. Congenital toxoplasmosis causes widespread calcification in contrast to the predominantly periventricular distribution of congenital cytomegalovirus infection. Both tuberous sclerosis and neurofibromatosis may be complicated by calcified cerebral abnormalities and another neurocutaneous syndrome, Sturge–Weber syndrome, may be identified by the unique double track linear calcification on skull radiography. Some slow-growing tumours such as craniopharyngioma may become calcified. The normal pineal gland may become calcified. Rett's syndrome, approximate incidence of 1:10 000–1:12 000 girls, is associated with loss of acquired speech and regression leading to stable mental handicap with some autistic-like features.

52. A – T; B – F; C – T; D – F; E – T

Maple syrup urine disease is an inborn error of metabolism. This aminoacidaemic disorder affects the metabolism of leucine, isoleucine and valine, resulting in high plasma and urine levels. The latter gives rise to its characteristic smell. Presentation is usually within the neonatal period with seizures, encephalopathy, hypoglycaemia and acidosis. Untreated infants deteriorate into a coma with apnoea and respiratory arrest. Milder variants have been described. Strict dietary control is necessary. Intercurrent illness associated with vomiting and dehydration may precipitate a crisis. Therefore fluid and dietary emergency plans need to be organised to prevent such an occurrence.

Hulse JA. Metabolic disorders. In: Clayden GS, Hawkins RL (eds). Treatment and prognosis in paediatrics. Heinemann, London. 1988:156.

53. A – T; B – T; C – F; D – T; E – T

Turner's syndrome comprises gonadal agenesis, absence of secondary sexual characteristics, short stature, webbing of the neck and inconsistent cardiac defects. The prevalence is 1:2000 live-born females but estimates suggest the diagnosis in 1% of spontaneous abortions. The karyotype of 45XO is due to loss of the paternally-derived X chromosome in 90%. DNA studies suggest all live-born cases have some degree of mosaicism which protects from abortion. Fetuses with cystic hygromata usually have hydrops fetalis (90%) and this is associated with a poor outcome. All forms of congenital heart disease are more common particularly aortic coarctation (30%) and left-sided valvular lesions. Visuospatial learning difficulties are common but intelligence is normal. Short stature is due to reduced intrauterine growth and subsequent reduced height velocity in childhood. There is no adolescent growth spurt. 20% enter puberty but only 1% complete it. Studies suggest improved growth with oxandrolone and growth hormone supplementation together in combination or singly. Oestrogens should be administered at puberty. Clinodactyly is an inconsistent feature of Down's syndrome.

Pearce JH. Turner's syndrome. Mat Child Health. 1992;12:365–9.

54. A – F; B – T; C – T; D – F; E – T

Necrotising enterocolitis is more common in preterm and growth-retarded infants but can occur spontaneously in term infants with no identified risk factors. The multifactorial aetiology includes mesenteric hypoperfusion due to asphyxia, hypovolaemia, use of indomethacin, patent ductus arteriosus plus 'gut stress' due to early feeds, particularly hyperosmolar feeds and infection. The presence and position of umbilical arterial catheters has not been reliably linked to necrotising enterocolitis. Clostridial isolates have been inconsistently detected in some cases. Hirschsprung's disease presenting as acute enterocolitis occurs. Clinical features include abdominal distension with nasogastric aspirates, collapse and metabolic acidosis with apnoea. Radiological features include fixed dilated oedematous loops of bowel; fluid levels; intramural gas (pneumatosis intestinalis); perforation and latterly, intrabiliary gas. 20% of infants require surgery. Mortality reaches 40% in some studies.

Simmer K, Roberts D. Neonatal disorders. In: Clayden GS, Hawkins RL (eds). Treatment and prognosis in paediatrics. Heinemann, London. 1988:16–7.

55. A – F; B – T; C – T; D – F; E – F

William's syndrome comprises: typical 'elfin' facies with upturned nose, low-set ears, prominent cheeks; cardiac defects particularly supravalvular aortic stenosis and developmental delay. It is also associated with hypercalcaemia. Other causes of hypercalcaemia include idiopathic, arising from increased sensitivity to vitamin D; vitamin D intoxication and primary hyperparathyroidism. Di George syndrome comprises thymic aplasia, T cell defects and absent parathyroid glands causing hypocalcaemia. Hypocalcaemia accompanies acute pancreatitis. Wilson's disease is an abnormality of copper metabolism.

Hulse JA. Metabolic disorders. In: Clayden GS, Hawkins RL (eds). Treatment and prognosis in paediatrics. Heinemann, London. 1988:165.

56. A – T; B – T; C – F; D – T; E – F

Many syndromes or inherited diseases are associated with deafness. They may cause both conductive and sensorineural deafness. Pendred's syndrome, incidence 2:100 000, is the association of deafness with hypothyroidism. Treacher–Collins syndrome is a cause of congenital conductive deafness associated with the classic unusual facies of mandibular facial dysostosis. Waardenburg's syndrome includes epicanthic folds, heterochromia iridium and a broad streak of white hair in the forelock. These changes may stem from abnormal neural crest cells. Usher's syndrome is the association of sensorineural deafness with retinitis pigmentosa. Hunter's syndrome is an X-linked mucopolysaccharidosis.

57. A – F; B – T; C – T; D – F; E – F

Preterm formula milks are modified by: increasing sodium content to counteract the preterm infant's increased renal leak; increased energy content and increased calcium/phosphate content to help reduce metabolic bone disease of prematurity. The majority of infants lose approximately 0.5 ml blood as gastrointestinal losses. In infants fed with milks containing cow's milk protein this loss may be increased. This may rarely be sufficient to produce melaena. The iron content of unmodified cow's milk contains less iron than formula milk as does breast milk. Semi-skimmed and skimmed milk are not recommended because of their limited energy content. Ordinary cow's milk is not recommended for those below one year of age as the amount of vitamin D and iron are reduced plus there is a risk of increased gastrointestinal blood loss.

Wharton B. Milk for babies and children. Br Med J. 1990;301:774–5.

58. A – T; B – F; C – F; D – T; E – T

Varicella is a common, highly infectious virus of the herpes family. Incubation period is 14–21 days accompanied by a short prodrome. The rash begins as macules progressing to papules, vesicles, pustules then crusting. Cases remain infectious until there are no new crops occurring. No part of the body is spared although trunk and covered areas are mainly affected. Haemorrhagic varicella may occur, particularly in the immunocompromised, leading to marked thrombocytopenia and poor outcome. Acute cerebellar ataxia, a post-infectious state, occurs as the rash is resolving. It is a mild cerebellitis which resolves in 2 weeks. Pneumonitis, myocarditis and secondary bacterial sepsis may occur. Varicella has been associated with Reye's syndrome. Congenital varicella infection can lead to limb deformities and cicatrial scarring. Neonatal varicella is associated with a significant mortality.

59. A – F; B – F; C – T; D – F; E – F

Constitutional delay in growth and puberty is one end of the normal
spectrum of pubertal development. It is much more common in boys.
Pubertal development is delayed, thus delaying the usual late male
pubertal growth spurt. Therefore the late childhood growth velocity
deceleration is prolonged. The result is a short boy compared to his
peers. There is often a positive family history. Characteristically there is
segmental disproportion with short spine and long legs. However, the
typical pattern of development (consonance) of puberty is not affected.
Dissonance of puberty points to a more sinister diagnosis. If untreated,
puberty and a slightly attenuated growth spurt will occur with epiphyseal
fusion occurring later than normal. However this diagnosis is associated
with considerable psychological problems. Oral oxandrolone, an
anabolic steroid, will institute an increase in growth whereas
intramuscular testosterone will induce both a growth spurt and
secondary sexual characteristics.

Stanhope R. Management of constitutional delay of growth and puberty. Growth
Matters. 1990;5:2–5.

60. A – F; B – T; C – F; D – T; E – F

Slipped femoral epiphyses occur in older children/adolescents resulting
in a painful hip with limited movement. An imbalance in growth
hormone and sex hormones may predispose to this diagnosis which may
be confirmed radiologically. 90% of children with hip pain and limp
have irritable hip (transient synovitis). This has a post-viral aetiology
and usually resolves with rest or, occasionally, traction. A small minority
may eventually progress to avascular necrosis of the femoral head
(Perthes' disease). This is usually in those aged 5 and above.
Malignancy, notably acute lymphoblastic leukaemia and metastatic
neuroblastoma, may cause a painful limp in this age group.
Osgood–Schlatter disease is a traction apophysitis causing knee pain on
quadriceps contraction. It does not cause a limp and is usually seen in
those aged 10–15 years, particularly boys.